RESISTANCE TRAINING EXERCISES

Fitness and Performance Exercises

for Strength, Stability and Mobility

RESISTANCE TRAINING EXERCISES

Fitness and Performance Exercises

for Strength, Stability and Mobility

Marina Aagaard, MFE

Aarhus, Denmark

aagaard | marina aagaard

RESISTANCE TRAINING EXERCISES

Fitness and Performance Exercises for Strength, Stability and Mobility

1. edition, 1. impression

ISBN 978-87-92693-52-5

Editor:	Marina Aagaard
Graphic design:	Marina Aagaard
Photographer (cover):	CPhotography, www.cphotography.com
	Cover model: Heidi Tang Moeller
Photographer:	Marina Aagaard, Henrik Elstrup
Printer:	Lulu.com
Printed in the US, 2010	

aagaard | marina aagaard

www.marinaaaagaard.dk

Contents

Preface

Welcome *to Resistance Training Exercises*. A comprehensive guide to resistance training exercises at all levels.

The book is intended for coaches, trainers, instructors, physiotherapists as well as physical education teachers and studens with some basic knowledge of physiology and training.
Many books provide the prerequisites for exercise selection and programme design. This book is dedicated to giving you as many exercises and variations as possible.

The book fills an important gap, as it presents exercises at all levels, from exercises used in rehabilitation and recreational exercises, all the way up to exercises used by Olympic athletes. This provides coaches, trainers, instructors and teachers with a meta-view of the wide range of exercises and variations and helps in selecting suitable exercises as well as progressing exercise programmes in better and more motivating ways.
Often, when you are in a certain sport or training milieu, you have a range of exercises that you and your peers before you have been using for years and keep coming back to.
However, there is a demand for a wider variety of exercises in order to provide mental and physical variation and stimulation to the people you coach, train and teach.

One important purpose of this book is to make it easier and more expedient to find the specific exercise you are looking for. It accomplishes this by bringing together a multitude of exercises from all over the world with bodyweight and different pieces of equipment in just one book.
The prime goal is to provide exercises for resistance training workouts, which are safe, specific, time-efficient and enjoyable for all involved.

I wish you good reading and good training.
Marina Aagaard, 2010

Aknowledgements

I am grateful for the many people who helped in making this book possible: My husband, family and friends for supporting and encouraging me.

Thanks to all of you who provided inspiration and feedback throughout the years, colleagues and students at the Academy of Coaching, Aalborg Sportshoejskole, colleagues and students at Aalborg University, professors and fellow students at The University of Southern Denmark, fellow intercontinental FIG coaches and friends at the Danish Gymnastics Federation.

Special thanks to Henriette Schaumburg-Müller and Alexander Benckendorff for reading and checking the English version of this book.

Special thanks to the fitness models, the energetic and patient trainers who helped in making this book come to life:
Diploma fitness coach Jacob Cornelius Hansen
Diploma strength training coach Morten Kirstein
Physiotherapist Heidi Tang Moeller
Diploma fitness coach Nicholas Krobath Olesen
Coach Mirela Ahmethodzic

Marina Aagaard, 2010

1 | How to Use This Book

Resistance Training Exercises is a comprehensive resource for coaches, trainers, instructors, physiotherapists and PE teachers. The exercises are for sports, gymnastics or general fitness and health, for individual exercise, partner exercise, small group exercise and group exercise.

All exercises are illustrated with photos and accompanied by descriptions and notes as well as suggestions for variations.

Some basic knowledge of anatomy, physiology and exercise science is needed to select, sequence and execute the exercises correctly. Do not progress without the help of a fitness professional, if you are unfamiliar with resistance training.

Important: All exercises are for healthy exercisers free from any serious or disabilitating disease, illness or ailments. Please consult your doctor before beginning these exercises.

Programme design – number of sets and repetitions, duration of rest-pauses and speed of movement – except for a few cases, is not discussed. This will vary with the goal of the exercise and the skill and strength of the exerciser. Other books cover these areas in detail.

The exercises are listed by muscle groups and in most instances after increasing level of difficulty. However, there are some exceptions, as many factors play a role.

The exercises are diverse, some are simple, some advanced. You must choose what is right for a given exerciser in a given situation.

The book contains exercises at all levels, from introductory to advanced, even Olympic, level. An advanced exerciser is a person, who is experienced, skilled and strong.

The weightlifting exercises of 'snatch' and 'clean and jerk', however, are not included. These exercises should form the basis of sports programmes, but they require more explanation and coaching than can be provided for in this book, so you are advised to contact a professional weightlifting instructor.

2 | Technique and safety

In order to maximize your workout benefit and minimize ineffecient use of your time or risk of injury, this chapter sums up the main points of proper exercise technique.

The exercise tables only list general and special points for exercise technique. In all exercises a **good posture is a prerequisite**: A strong and stable body with stabilizing core muscles.

Depending on the exercise, whether being an isolation exercise or compound exercise, you focus on either one primary muscle or a muscle group or a number of muscles in one controlled movement.

You should *avoid unwanted co-movements, such as the head and shoulder girdle dropping forward, excessive arching or hunching of the lower back, and locking of the knees or elbows.*

Breathing should be deep abdominal breathing using the diaphragm. Inhale through the nose and exhale through the nose or mouth. During all exercises keep breathing deeply, this will increase the energy and enhance the workout.

The typical resistance training breathing pattern is biomechanical breathing:
Inhale on the eccentric phase of the exercise and exhale on the concentric phase for greater force production.

Anatomical breathing: You inhale when you extend your back, opening up your ribcage allowing for more air into the lungs and exhale when you bend the torso, reducing space for air.

The exercises should be preceeded by a warm-up of 5-20 minutes depending of the intensity and duration of the workout.

Programme design will vary with the goal of the exercise and the skill and strength level of the exerciser. However, for general fitness 1-3 sets of 8-12 repetitions of 8-10 exercises for major muscle groups are appropriate.

The exercise tempo should be moderate and rest-pauses around ½-2 minutes. Exercise should be followed by a cooldown, eg. walk round the room, of 3-5 minutes depending of the intensity and the exerciser. Include relevant stretches as needed.

Basic posture

Initiate all workouts and exercises with a good posture: The prerequisite for optimal results.

Front view: Imagine a plumb line through the middle of the body. Head and neck, shoulders and hips should form a symmetrical image around this line.

Side view: Image a plumb line passing through the ear, shoulder, hip, knee and ankle (right in front of the outer malleol bone).

If you see significant deviations from this, you need to correct the posture or do some exercises, which will help you obtain a better posture. In some instances you need to have a physiotherapist perform relevant testing and provide the necessary corrective exercises.

Focus points standing starting position:

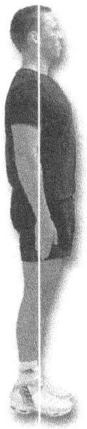

- Legs together or hip- or shoulder-width apart.
- Feet forward or a little outward in a natural outward rotation.
- Feet are firmly positioned with the weight evenly distributed across the foot; keep the heel and toes on the ground.
- Knees are aligned with feet; knee aligned with the second toe.
- Knees are relaxed, not locked, hyperextended, or overly flexed.
- Pelvis is in a neutral position.
- Transversus abdominis contracts as needed to stabilize the spine.
- The spine is in neutral position with a natural curve.
- Shoulder blades are in neutral.
- Shoulders are lowered and level.
- Neck is in neutral position.
- Tongue rests in the roof of the mouth behind the front teeth.

Guidelines Elastic Resistance Training

Improve your elastic resistance training and avoid accidents by observing these precautions:

- Choose a suitable resistance. If you are unable to complete 8-12 repetitions, you should initially choose a lighter elastic band.
- Always check your equipment for wear and tear. Throw away broken bands and tubes. Elastic bands etc. should not be exposed to direct sunlight or water.
- Always check the joints between the elastic materials and the handles or straps.
- Always check that bindings and straps are firmly secured before starting the exercise.
- Elastic tubes – and bands – can be tied together and used as one piece of equipment, however, they are difficult to untie, so other alternatives are preferred.
- Do not wear rings, watches or jewellery when using elastic equipment.
- Do not press your fingers or nails into the elastic material.
- Do not maximally stretch a cold piece of elastic material to its maximum, warm it up a little, use exercises with a smaller range of motion.
- Do not stretch rubberbands and tubing over 2-3 times resting length.
- Do not stretch the resistance band over 3-5 times resting length (depending on brand).
- Always control the exercise, the pull of the elastic band, also during the eccentric phase.
- Protect you eyes. When you have checked the binding and exercise technique, look away from, do not look directly at, the elastic piece of equipment.
- The pull of the elastic piece of equipment should be in the direct opposite direction of the muscle (fibers) you wish to work.

Tube and band bindings

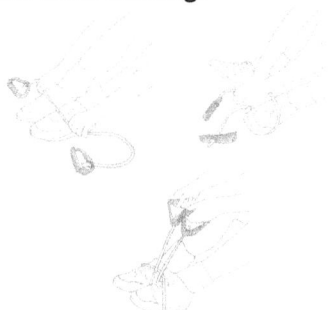

Example of foot binding for securing tube around the feet. 1) Over the feet, 2) under the feet, and, 3) up between the feet

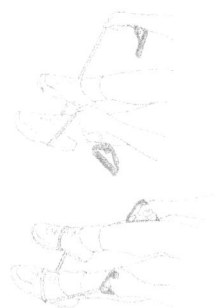

Binding with an ekstra ½ loop – tightens the tube; 1) under, 2) over, 3) under.

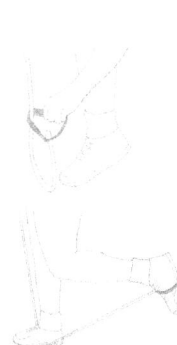

Single loop for securing the tube around the foot.

Guidelines Free Weight Resistance Training

Improve your free weight exercise programme and avoid accidents by observing these simple precautions:

- Barbells and adjustable dumbbells: Equal load at both sides – and both dumbbells.
- Barbells and adjustable dumbbells: Secure the weight plates with a collar or clamp.
- Dumbbells in more parts: Check that the dumbbell is in one piece and the dumbbell weight plates are securely fastened.
- Barbells: Hold the bar with an even grip with both hands, so the bar is in balance.
- Barbells and dumbbells: Lift with a firm, closed grip, four fingers around the bar and the thumb closing. Do not use an *open* or *false grip* with all five fingers on one side, as you risk the weight falling from your hands onto your torso or limbs.
- Lift with proper lifting technique.
- Pay attention. Be careful not to accidentally drop barbells, dumbbells or weight plates.
- Put back the dumbbells in the rack, in pairs in their proper spot.
- Do not drop dumbbells or barbells, it is noisy and damages the dumbbells and flooring. Exception: When weightlifting in a weightlifting room with special flooring.

Correct lifting technique is: The right technique according to the exercise in question, but also when transporting, moving, dumbbells, bars and other equipment:

- Get close to the equipment.
- Stand with feet firmly on the floor.
- Lift with a firm closed grip.
- Hold your wrists neutral.
- Lift with your legs and arms, not just the back.
- Lift and carry the equipment close to your body.
- When lifting and turning, turn the whole body, not just the spine.

3 | Shoulder Exercises

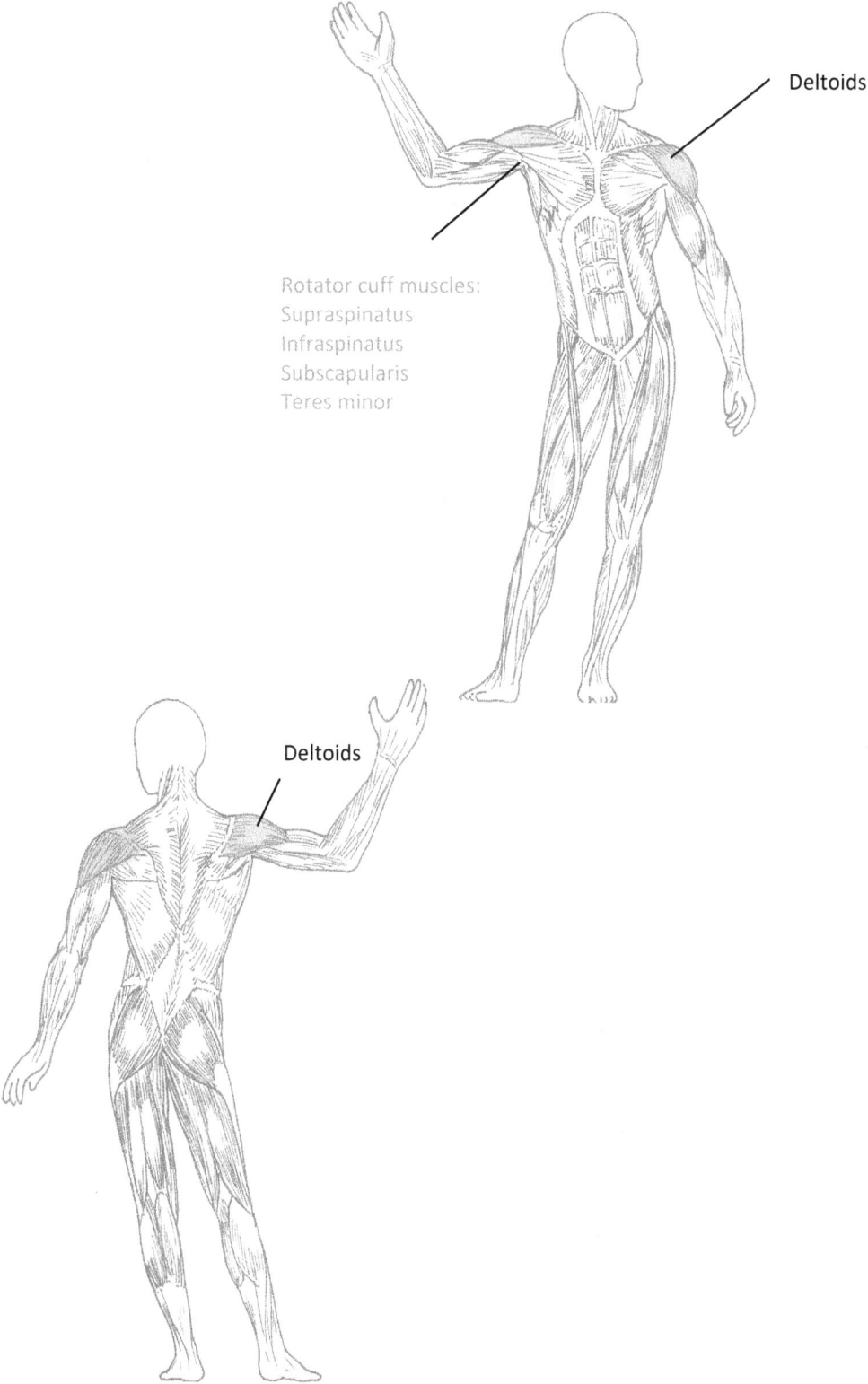

Deltoids

Rotator cuff muscles:
Supraspinatus
Infraspinatus
Subscapularis
Teres minor

Deltoids

EXERCISE	TECHNIQUE

FRONT RAISE

Primary muscles:
Anterior deltoid

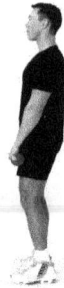

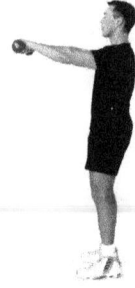

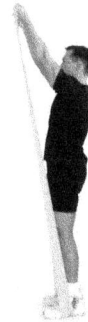

**HIGH FRONT RAISE
WITH RESISTANCE BAND**

Primary muscles:
Anterior deltoid

SHOULDER PRESS

Primary muscles:
Anterior and medial
deltoid

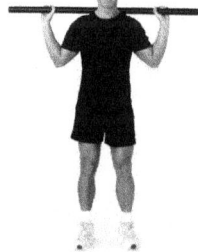

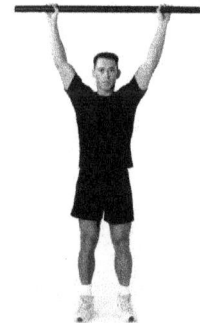

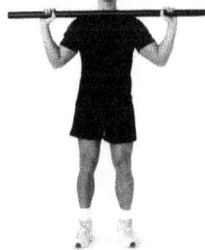

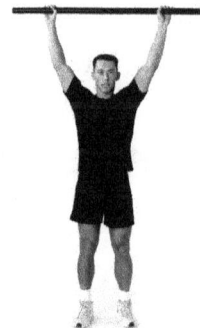

**MILITARY PRESS
(FRONT PRESS)**

Primary muscles:
Anterior and medial
deltoid

Standing. Dumbbells, tube or band in hands. Arms at sides or in front of thighs. Raise arm(s) in front of the body to horizontal. Lower with control.	Core muscles stabilize. In this exercise there is a tendency to arch the back, and pull with the lower back. Avoid this, lift with control.	Different body/leg position. Standing, sitting, kneeling. Uni- or bilateral, alternating. Straight or bent arms (elbows). Over-, under-, neutral grip. Dumbbells, barbell, tube, band, medicine ball. **ONE DUMBBELL FRONT RAISE** Hands together lifting one dumbbell.
Standing. Band anchored under foot/feet. Held by the hands. Arms at sides or in front of the thighs. Palms face each other. Raise arm(s) in front of the body towards vertical position. Lower with control.	Core muscles stabilize. In this exercise there is a tendency to arch and pull with the lower back. Avoid this. Avoid shoulder impingement: Throughout exercise, or when approaching horizontal, turn palms towards each other.	Different body/leg position. Standing, sitting, kneeling. Unilateral, bilateral or alternating. Straight or bent arms (elbows). Dumbbells, band.
Standing. Elbows bent. Hands by the shoulders. With a barbell behind the head. Overhand wide grip (control: when the upper arms are horizontal, the forearms are vertical). Push arms upwards to vertical. Lower, until the upper arms come close to sides of torso.	May be hard on the shoulders especially with a limited ROM in the shoulders. Note: Above horizontal there is risk of shoulder impingement. Neutral grip is preferred. Full Range of Motion: Upper arms by the sides of the torso up to vertical position.	Different body/leg position. Standing, sitting, kneeling. Overhand or neutral grip (with dumbbells or special bar). One or both arms. Dumbbells, barbell, tube, band, medicine ball or one dumbbell.
Standing. Shoulder press with barbell in front of the neck. Arms bent. Hands at shoulder level. Overhand wide grip (when upper arms are in horizontal, forearms are vertical). Press arms up. Lower, until the upper arms touch the side of body.	May be hard on the shoulders especially with a limited ROM in the shoulders. Note: Above horizontal there is risk of shoulder impingement. Neutral grip is preferred. Full Range of Motion: Upper arms by the side of the body to vertical position.	Different body/leg position. Standing, sitting, kneeling. Overhand or neutral grip. Shoulder-width grip, elbows forward: focus anterior deltoids and chest. Wide grip, elbows out, focus deltoids, anterior and medial part. Dumbbells, tube or band.

EXERCISE	TECHNIQUE

SHOULDER PRESS WITH DUMBBELLS (DUMBELL PRESS)

Primary muscles: Anterior and medial deltoid

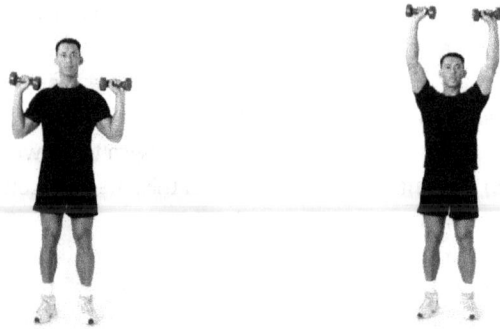

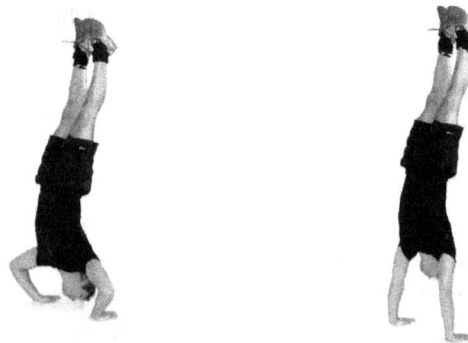

PUSHING GEORGIA AWAY

Primary muscles: Anterior and medial deltoid

PUSH PRESS

Primary muscles: Anterior and medial deltoid, and hips and legs

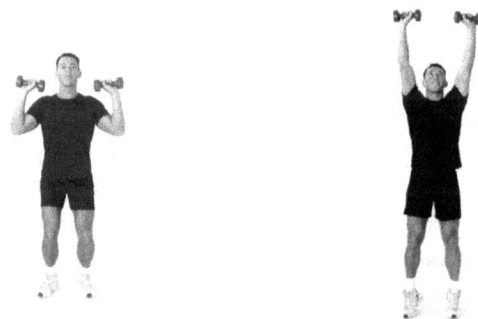

CURL TO PRESS

Primary muscles: Biceps brachii, brachialis, anterior and medial deltoid

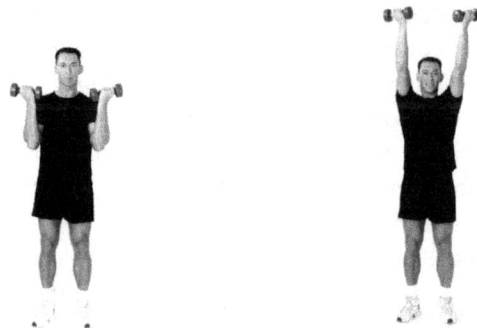

Standing. Shoulder press with dumbbells. Start and finish with the hands by the shoulders. Push the arms up into vertical position. Do not hyperextend, lock, the elbows. Lower until the upper arms are close to the sides of the torso.	May be hard on the shoulders especially with a limited ROM in the shoulders. Note: Above horizontal there is risk of shoulder impingement. Neutral grip is preferred. Full Range of Motion: Upper arms by the side of the body is the starting position.	Different body/leg position. Standing, sitting, kneeling. Unilateral, bilateral, alternating. Over-, under-, neutral grip. Dumbbells, tube, band.
Standing, handstand. Hands wider than shoulder-width apart. Body is vertical with legs up. Legs can be unsupported or supported by a wall or a partner. Arms push off to a shoulder press with the body as resistance.	Advanced exercise. You have to have excellent core control and balance as well as shoulder strength in order to execute this exercise.	With or without support for the legs (by wall or partner).
Standing. Shoulder press with power. Starting position as shoulder press with dumbbells. Bend legs fast and then extend forcefully, so the legs and torso power the arms and shoulders to forcefully push the dumb-bells upwards. Lower with control.	Advanced exercise. This exercise is mostly used for lifting heavier dumbbells, than can be lifted without the 'push'.	Different leg position.
Standing. The exercise starts like a biceps curl – arms at sides and bend the elbows – but from top position continue upwards into a shoulder press with an underhand grip. Lower back down.	Combination exercise.	Different leg position. Dumbbells, barbell, tube or band.

EXERCISE	TECHNIQUE

ARNOLD PRESS

Primary muscles:
Anterior and medial
deltoid

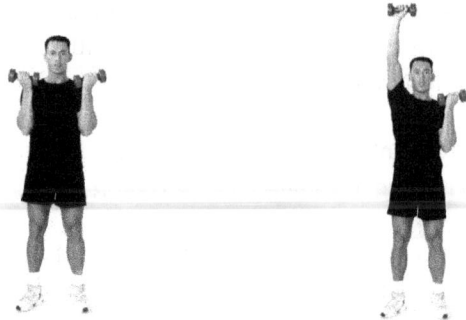

CLEAN'N'PRESS

Primary muscles:
Biceps brachii, brachialis,
anterior and medial
deltoid

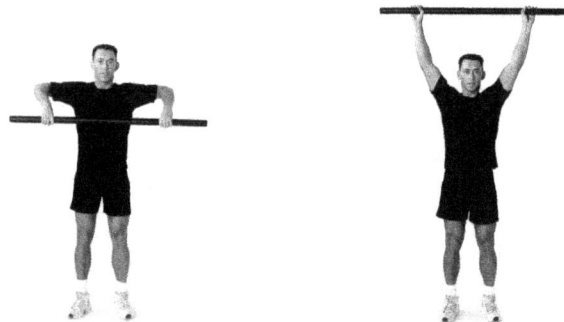

UPRIGHT ROWING

Primary muscles:
Anterior and medial deltoid,
biceps brachii

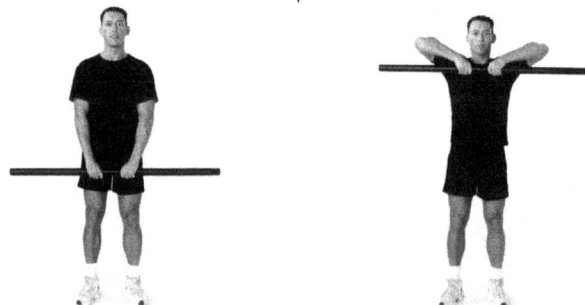

AROUND THE WORLD

Primary muscles:
Deltoids, rotator cuff

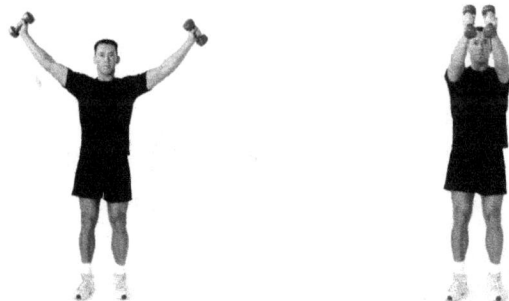

Standing. The arms are bent in front of the body, as in biceps curl top position. Palms face the torso. Dumbbells in hands. From here press one arm upwards into vertical shoulder press, while the arm rotates, so the palm faces forward. Lower back down and repeat with opposite arm.	In top position the arms is rotated, which may cause shoulder impingement. The arm is straight, but not locked, hyperextended, the elbow is 'relaxed'.	Different leg position. Standing, sitting, kneeling. Unilateral, bilateral, alternating. With dumbbells, tube or band.
Standing 'upright rowing' with a wide grip. From top position continue up into shoulder press with an overhand grip. As in cleans you use the shoulders and trapezius to accellerate the barbell upwards. Lower with control the same way down.	Combination exercise.	Different leg position. With dumbbells, barbell, tube or band. **REVERSE BICEPS CURL TO PRESS** Hands shoulder-width apart. Biceps curl with overhand grip continue into shoulderpres.
Standing. Narrow overhand grip on barbell, in front of the body. Pull upwards, the elbows lead the way, so they are slightly higher than the hands, which stop under the chin (or at chest height to limit range of motion). Avoid bending the wrists. Lower with control.	Note: May cause shoulder impingement; stop when elbows are at or below shoulder level. When using a barbell, you find 'narrow grip' by grasping the middle of the barbell, putting the thumbs together, and then back around the barbell. They should not rest on the barbell.	Different body/leg position. Standing, sitting, kneeling. Unilateral, bilateral, alternating. With dumbbells, tube or band. **UPRIGHT ROWING, WIDE** Wide overhand grip. Barbell only to chestheight (to avoid shoulder impingement).
Standing. The arms at sides, the dumbbells in hands. The arms make a circle, outwards and upwards, in the frontal plane, up over the head (above shoulder level turn the palms upwards). Then lower the arms down in front of the torso back to starting position.	Helps in increasing shoulder range of motion. Great for variety. The exercise can be performed supine for a different effect.	Different body/leg position. Standing, sitting, lying. On floor, bench or ball. Unilateral, bilateral. The arms can be lowered the same way they came up, as a side lateral variation. All of the exercise in the frontal plane.

EXERCISE	TECHNIQUE

(SIDE) LATERAL RAISE

Primary muscles:
Medial deltoid

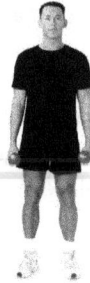

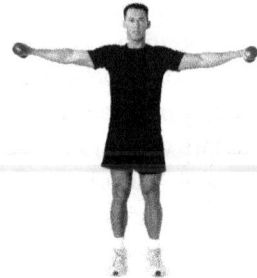

**REVERSE OVERHEAD
SIDE LATERALS**

Primary muscles:
Anterior and medial deltoid

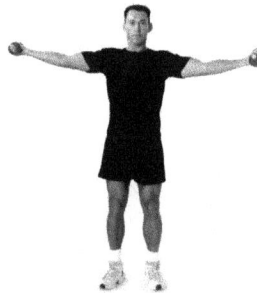

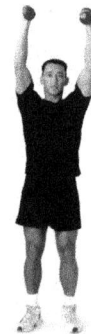

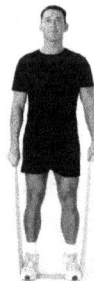

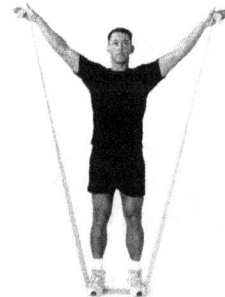

**LATERAL RAISE, HIGH,
WITH RESISTANCE BAND**

Primary muscles:
Anterior and medial deltoid

**DIAGONAL
FRONTAL RAISE**

Primary muscles:
Deltoids, supraspinatus

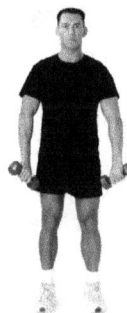

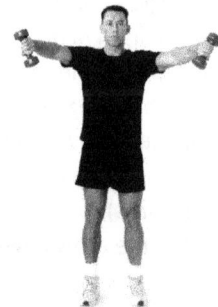

Standing. Arms are straight, but not hypextended, at sides or in front of the body. Raise the arms to the side, to horizontal. Lower. Lift with the shoulders without unwanted movement in the lower back. Do not use a weight belt, the core muscles should stabilize.	Main exercise for targeting the middle part of the deltoids. Tip: You can lean the body a couple of degrees forward, the arms still straight to the side. Not recommended for general fitness, it increases the load on the lower back. Arms straight, but not hyper-extended, elbows 'relaxed'.	Different leg position. Standing, sitting, kneeling. Unilateral, bilateral. Straight or bent arms. If the dumbbells are very heavy bend the arms. Over-, under-, neutral grip. Dumbbells, barbell, tube, band.
Standing. Arms straight to the side in horizontal plane. The palms face upwards, underhand grip on dumbbells. From here lift the arms up into vertical, upper arms by the side of the head. Lower the arms back to horizontal.	The palms face upwards throughout the movement. The arms are straight, but not hyperextended, elbows are 'relaxed'.	Different body/leg position. Standing, sitting, kneeling. Unilateral, bilateral.
Standing. Straight arms at sides or together in front of the body. Palms towards torso, band around hands. Band is anchored under the feet. Raise the arms in frontal plane, to the side, up past horizontal. The palms turn forward during the movement. Lower.	Functional exercise with a large range of motion. The are arms straight, but not hyperextended, elbows are 'relaxed'.	Different leg position. Unilateral, bilateral. Straight or bent arms.
Standing. Arms at sides of the torso or in front of thighs. Overhand grip on dumbbells, band or tube. Raise arms diagonally up and outwards to horizontal. Lower.	If you experience impingement symptoms, do not perform this exercise past your pain level. Variation: Hands face slightly downwards as if pouring water from a bottle.	Different body/leg position. Standing, sitting, kneeling. Unilateral, bilateral. With dumbbells, tube or band.

**REAR LATERAL RAISE
UNILATERAL
WITH TUBE OR BAND**

Primary muscles:
Medial deltoid

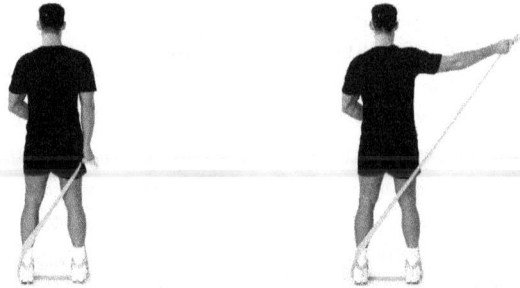

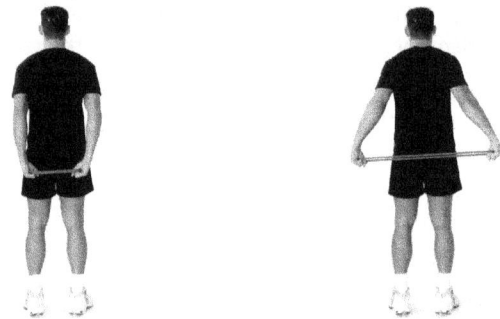

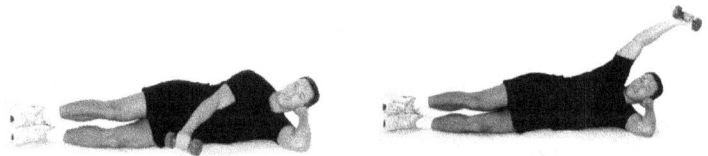

**REAR LATERAL RAISE
BILATERAL
WITH RUBBERBAND**

Primary muscles:
Medial deltoid

**AROUND THE WORLD
SIDELYING**

Primary muscles:
Medial deltoid

**LATERAL RAISE,
SIDELYING**

Primary muscles:
Medial deltoid,
supraspinatus

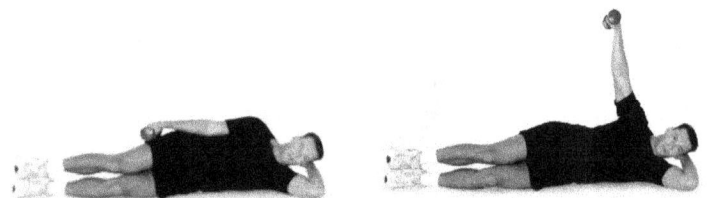

TECHNIQUE	NOTES	VARIATION
Standing. Tube or band under opposite foot, behind the body. Resistance band in hand. Arm down at the side of body. Palm is facing downwards. Raise arm in frontal plane, to the side, up to horizontal. Lower.	The pull is slightly different when the resistance comes straight from the side. Contract the core muscles to stabilize the body. Arm straight, but not hyper-extended, elbow is 'relaxed'.	Different leg position. With tube or band.
Standing. The arms behind the body, palms towards each other, holding exercise band. Lift the arms to the side, away from each other, in frontal plane. Return with control.	Contract the core muscles to stabilize the body. Small range of motion. The arms are extended, but not locked, elbows are 'relaxed'.	Different leg position. With tube or band.
Sidelying. Top arm down by the side of the body. Palm forward. Lift arm laterally up to vertical, then lower the arm past the head (close to the ear). Arm moves in a semi-circle, in the horizontal plane in front of the body, back to starting position.	Arm is straight, but not locked, hyperextended, elbow is 'relaxed'. Note, that the arm rotates during the movement to avoid shoulder impingement.	Different leg position. On floor, bench or ball.
Sidelying. Top arm down at the side of the body or right in front of leg. Overhand grip on dumbbell. Lift arm up almost to vertical position. Lower.	Arm is straight, but not locked, hyperextended, elbow is 'relaxed'.	Different body position. On floor, bench or ball.

EXERCISE	TECHNIQUE

**SHOULDER EXTENSION
PRONE**

Primary muscles:
Posterior deltoid,
triceps brachii

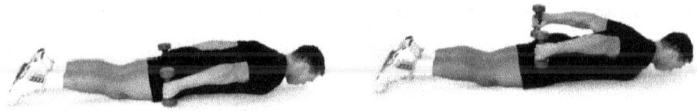

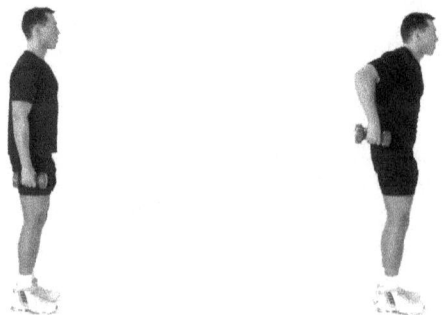

BACK FLY, SIDELYING

Primary muscles:
Posterior deltoid

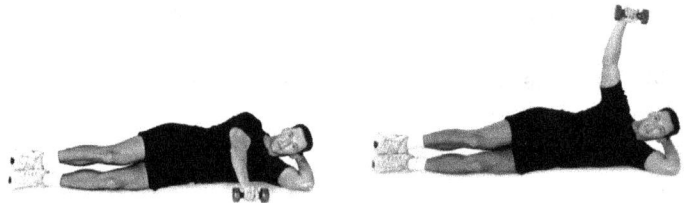

**BACK FLY
WITH BODYBAR**

Primary muscles:
Posterior deltoid,
rhomboids

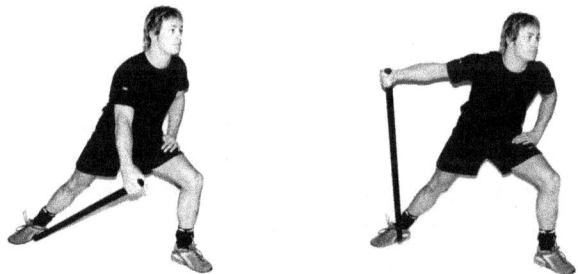

**SHOULDER EXTENSION,
BENT ARMS**

Primary muscles:
Posterior deltoid,
triceps brachii

TECHNIQUE	NOTES	VARIATION
Prone. Arms down at sides. Lift the arms straight upwards in sagittal plane. Lower, but stop just before the arms rest on the floor.	On a bench or ball the range of motion can be larger, which is preferable The arms/elbows are kept straight.	Different leg position. The angle of the arms to the torso may vary. One or both arms. On floor, ball or bench. With or without resistance.
Sidelying. Top arm straight and in front of the torso (90 degree angle). Overhand grip on dumbbell. Lift the arm up close to vertical position. Lower with control.	A different load through the range of motion compared to standing back fly. Arm/elbow is kept straight.	Different body position. On floor, bench or ball.
Standing. Legs are staggered. The body is leaning forward with the free hand on the thigh. Bodybar is supported by the inside of the foot of the back leg. The arm at the same side holds the bodybar. Lift the arm backwards in a semi-circular motion from the front of the body out and up.	Contract the core muscles to stabilize the body. Elbow is slightly bent. Avoid hyperextending the elbow in top position.	Different body position.
Standing. Straight arms down at sides or just behind the body. Lift the arms straight up/back In the sagittal plane. During the lift bend the arms. Lower with control.	Neck in neutral position: Ears above the shoulders. (In the photo the head has come slightly forward).	Different leg position. One or both arms. Bent or straight the arms. Over-, under-, neutral grip. Dumbbells, barbell, tube or band.

EXERCISE	TECHNIQUE

SHOULDER EXTENSION

Primary muscles:
Posterior deltoid,
triceps brachii

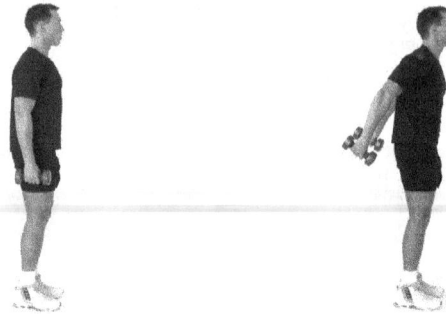

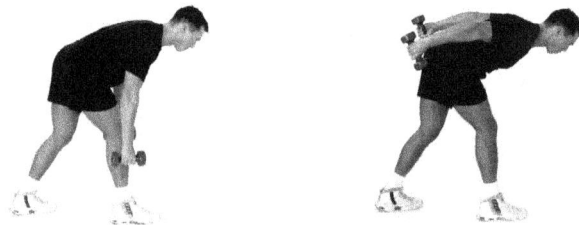

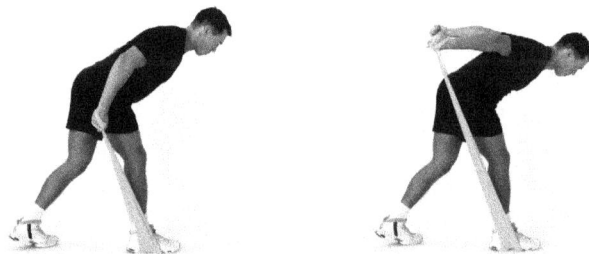

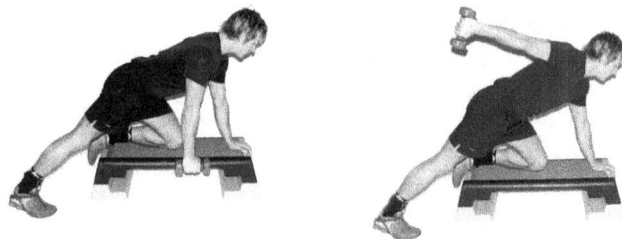

**SHOULDER EXTENSION
BENT-OVER**

Primary muscles:
Posterior deltoid,
triceps brachii

**SHOULDER EXTENSION
BENT-OVER
WITH RESISTANCE BAND**

Primary muscles:
Posterior deltoid,
triceps brachii

**SHOULDER EXTENSION,
UNILATERAL,
KNEELING**

Primary muscles:
Posterior deltoid,
triceps brachii

Standing. Arms down by the side. Lift arms straight back In the sagittal plane. Lift with the shoulders with no unwanted movement of the torso. Lower. Stop, while arms are just behind the body, before vertical position.	Contract the core muscles to stabilize the body. Neck in neutral position. The arms/elbows are kept straight.	Different body/leg position. Unilateral, bilateral. Straight or bent arms. Over-, under-, neutral grip. With dumbbells, barbell, tube, band.
Standing. Forward lean. Arms down a little behind vertical position. Lift the arms straight back and upwards in the sagittal plane. Lift with the shoulders without unwanted movement of the torso. Lower, stop just before vertical position.	Contract the core muscles to stabilize the body. Beginners and people with back problems should perform the exercise with only one arm, while the other is supported on the thigh. The elbows are kept straight.	Different body/leg position. Unilateral, bilateral. With or without support. Straight or bent arms. Over-, under-, neutral grip. Dumbbells, barbell, tube, band.
Standing. Forward lean. The arms down, close to vertical position. Lift the arms back in the sagittal plane. Lift with the shoulders with no unwanted movement of the torso. Lower to vertical, stop, while there is still tension in the band.	Contract the core muscles to stabilize the body. Neck in neutral position. The arms/elbows are kept straight.	Different body/leg position. Unilateral, bilateral. Straight or bent arms. Over-, under-, neutral grip. With tube or band.
Kneeling. One knee on bench. Body is leaning forward. Hand of the same side on the bench. Working arm down. Lift arm straight back In the sagittal plane. Lift with shoulder with no unwanted movement of the back. Lower, stop just before the arm reaches vertical position.	Contract the core muscles to stabilize the body. Neck in neutral position. Arm/elbow is kept straight.	Different body/leg position. Unilateral, bilateral. With or without support. Straight or bent arms. Over-, under-, neutral grip.

EXERCISE	TECHNIQUE

BACK FLYS,
PRONE
(PRONE REVERSE FLYS)

Primary muscles:
Posterior deltoid,
rhomboids, middle trapezius

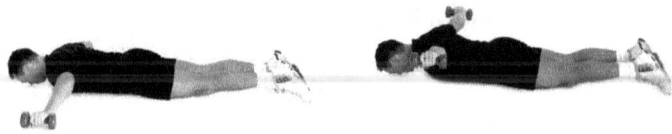

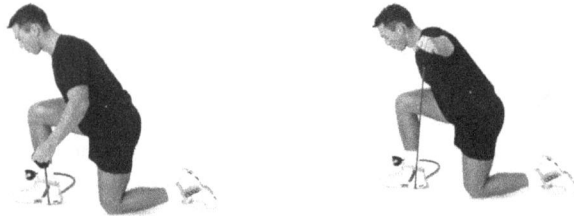

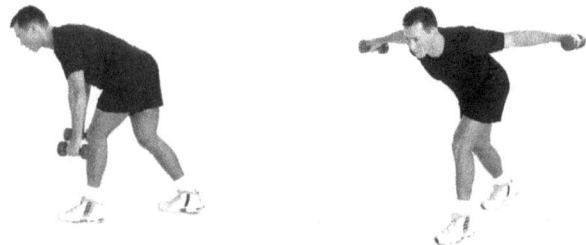

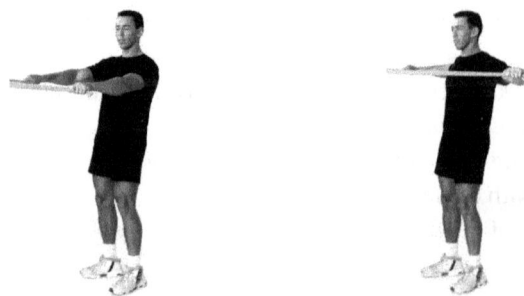

BACK FLYS, UNILATERAL,
KNEELING
WITH TUBE

Primary muscles:
Posterior deltoid,
rhomboids, middle trapezius

BACK FLYS,
WITH FORWARD LEAN
(REVERSE FLYS)

Primary muscles:
Posterior deltoid,
rhomboids, middle trapezius

BACK FLYS, STANDING
(REVERSE FLYS)
WITH TUBE/BAND

Primary muscles:
Posterior deltoid,
rhomboids, middle trapezius

Prone. The arms straight to the side. Dumbbells in hands, overhand grip. Lift arms upwards in the horizontal plane. In top position adduct the shoulder blades. Lower.	An important postural exercise. On a bench or ball the range of motion is greater, which is preferable.	One or both arms. With or without resistance. On floor, ball or bench. **AT DIFFERENT ANGLES** Arms extended over the head, 45° up and out, 45° down and out, and all angles in between.
Kneeling. Forward lean. Arms down. Tube/band in hand. Tube/band anchored under the front foot. Lift the arm straight outwards in a bent-over lateral raise. In top position adduct the shoulder blade. Lower with control.	Contract the core muscles to stabilize the body.	Different body/leg position. Unilateral, bilateral. With or without support. Straight or bent arms. Over-, under-, neutral grip. With dumbbells, barbell, tube, band.
Standing. Forward lean. Arms down in front of the body. Dumbbells in the hands. Lift the arms straight out and upwards past horizontal. Lower with control	An important postural exercise. First part of the exercise involves the back of the shoulders, the last part, when the shoulder blades are adducted, the rhomboids and middle trapezius.	Different body/leg position. With or without support. One or both arms With dumbbells, barbell, tube or band.
Standing. The arms straight in front of the body. Elbows slightly bent. The hands hold tube or band, which is anchored by a wall bar (or partner) in front of the body. Pull the arms outwards and backwards in horizontal plane. Resist the return movement.	An important exercise for good posture. First part of the exercise involves the back of the shoulder, the last part, when the shoulder blades are adducted, the rhomboids and middle trapezius.	Different leg position. One or both arms. Bent or straight arms. Overhand grip or neutral grip.

EXERCISE	TECHNIQUE

**SHOULDER UNILATERAL
LATERAL ROTATION,
SIDELYING**

Primary muscles:
Infraspinatus

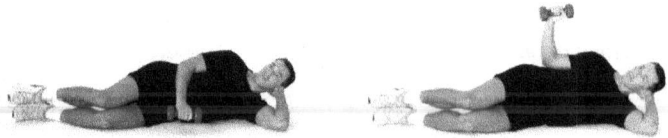

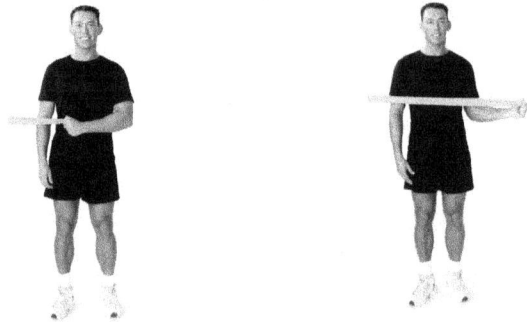

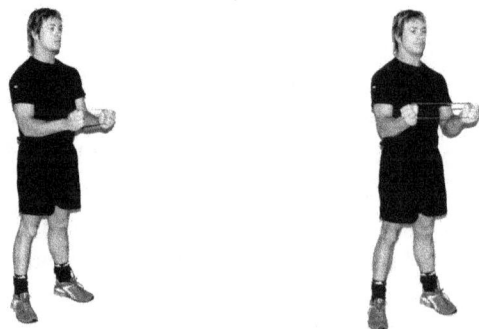

**SHOULDER UNILATERAL
LATERAL ROTATION, LOW
STANDING**

Primary muscles:
Infraspinatus

**SHOULDER UNILATERAL
LATERAL ROTATION, HIGH
STANDING**

Primary muscles:
Teres minor

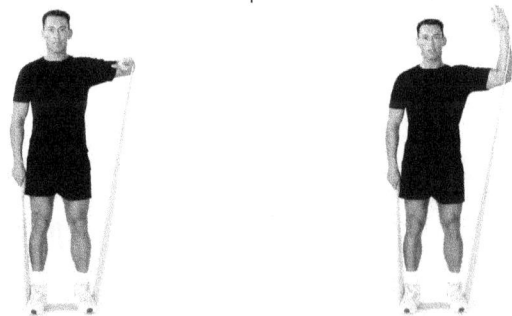

**SHOULDER
LATERAL ROTATION, LOW
STANDING**

Primary muscles:
Infraspinatus

Sidelying. Upper arm close to the body, elbow bent 90 degrees, the forearm in horizontal position. Elbow is close to the hip. Rotate the arm outwards and upwards, without the elbow moving.	Important shoulder stability exercise. Elbow must remain in place near the hip. If the elbow slides back and forth, the larger, outer muscles are taking over.	One or both arms. With or without resistance. On floor, ball or bench.
Standing. Upper arm close to the body, the arm is bent 90 degrees, the forearm in horizontal position. The resistance band is fixed to the side of the body at the opposite side. Band in hand. Rotate the arm outward, without the elbow moving. Return with control.	Important shoulder stability exercise. Elbow must stay in place, the upper arm close to the torso. If the elbow moves, the larger, outer muscles are taking over.	Different leg position. One or both arms. With rubberband, tube or band.
Standing. The band is anchored under the feet. Upper arm is in horizontal position. The elbow is bent 90 degrees, the forearm is in horizontal. Rotate the arm from horizontal to vertical and back down. The forearm may move below horizontal.	Important shoulder stability exercise. Elbow should stay in place, the arm around shoulderheight. If the elbow moves, the larger, outer muscles are taking over.	Different body/leg position. Shoulder angle may vary. Arm diagonal in front of the body (50-70 degrees). One or both arms. With tube or band.
Standing. Upper arms at sides, the arms bent 90 degrees, the forearms are in horizontal plane. The palms face each other. Resistance band around the hands. Rotate both arms outwards without the elbows moving. Return with control.	Shoulder stability exercise. Elbows should stay in place, upper arms close to the torso. If the elbows move, the larger, outer muscles are taking over.	Different leg position. One or both arms. With rubberband, tube or band.

**SHOULDER UNILATERAL
MEDIAL ROTATION,
SIDELYING**

Primary muscles:
Subscapularis

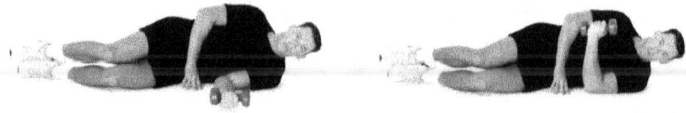

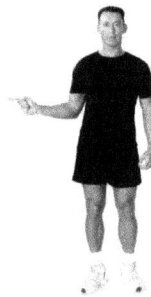

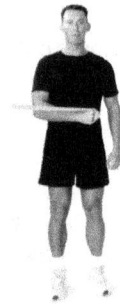

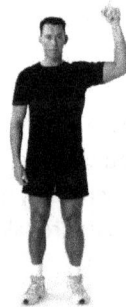

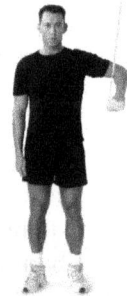

**SHOULDER UNILATERAL
MEDIAL ROTATION, LOW
STANDING**

Primary muscles:
Subscapularis

**SHOULDER UNILATERAL
MEDIAL ROTATION, HIGH
STANDING**

Primary muscles:
Subscapularis

**SHOULDERCIRCLES
OVER THE HEAD**

Primary muscles:
Deltoids androtator cuff

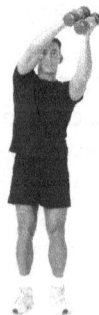

Sidelying (on bench or ball). Lower arm is bent 90 degrees and close to the body. Dumbbell in hand. Elbow is close to the hip – if you are on the floor, the elbow is just above the floor. Rotate the arm inwards (upwards) without the elbow moving. Lower with control.	Important shoulder stability exercise. Elbow should stay in place, the upper arm close to the torso. If the elbow moves, the larger, outer muscles are taking over.	One or both arms. On floor, ball or bench.
Standing. Upper arm close to the body, arm bent 90 degrees, forearm in horizontal. The palm faces upwards or inwards. Resistance band in hand. Rotate arm inwards without the elbow moving. Return with control.	Important shoulder stability exercise. Elbow should stay in place, the upper arm close to the torso. If the elbow moves, the larger, outer muscles are taking over.	Different leg position. With rubberband, tube or band.
Standing. Upper arm in horizontal. Elbow bent 90 degrees. Rotate forearms from vertical downwards to vertical. Resist return movement upwards.	Important shoulder stability exercise. Elbow should stay in place, the upper arm in horizontal. If the elbow moves, the larger, outer muscles are taking over.	Different leg/body position. One or both arms. With tube or band.
Standing. Both arms are extended over the head. The hands hold one dumbbell. The arms make circles above the head. Contract the core muscles to keep the body stable.	Core exercise. The arms are slightly bent or straight, not hyperextended, elbows are 'relaxed'.	Different leg position. One or both arms. Dumbbell, medicine ball or tornado ball (medicine ball on a rope).

EXERCISE	TECHNIQUE

REVERSE WOOD CHOP

Primary muscles:
Posterior deltoid,
rhomboids, rotators

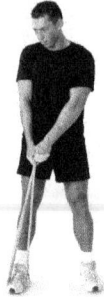

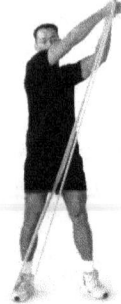

**SHOULDER ROTATION AND
PRESS WITH BARBELL
(CUBAN PRESS)**

Primary muscles:
Deltoids, teres minor

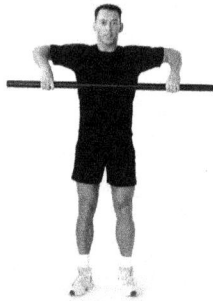

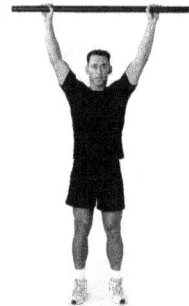

SHOULDER CIRCLES

Primary muscles:
Deltoids, rotator cuff

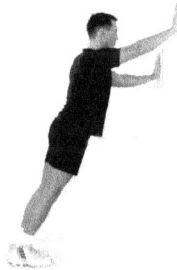

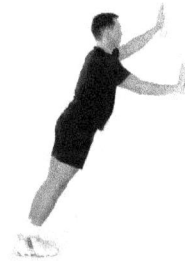

**SHOULDER
LATERAL ROTATION
STANDING, FORWARD LEAN**

Primary muscles:
Infraspinatus

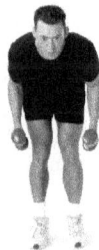

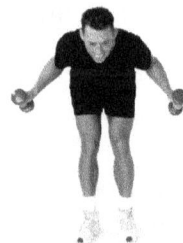

Standing. Both hands in front of the body, down to one side. Tube or band anchored under foot or wall bar. Pull arms pull diagonally upwards in front of the body to a point above the opposite shoulder. Lower.	Functional exercise. The opposite movement of woodchopping; lifting the axe.	Unilateral, bilateral. With or without torso rotation. With tube or band.
Standing. Barbell in hands, wide overhand grip. Upper arms in horizontal, forearms down, vertical. Forearms rotate upwards to vertical, then press barbell up with a shoulder press. Lower and rotate back down.	May be hard on the shoulders. Not recommended for general fitness. For advanced exercises.	Different leg position. One or both arms. With dumbbells or barbell.
Standing. Hands against wall (or kneeling with the hands on the floor). Hands on pieces of cloth or carpet or similar. The hands make small or large circles. The hands do not lift from the surface. Put more or less body weight into the movement (load).	Closed-chain exercise for rehabilitation of the shoulder. Also for preventive training in traditional workouts.	One or both arms. Body angle may vary.
Standing. Forward lean. Arms bent 90 degrees. Dumbbells in hands. Elbows are held in place, at sides of the torso. Rotate the arms out and back. Lower back with control.	Contract the core muscles to stabilize the body.	Different body/leg position.

EXERCISE	TECHNIQUE

**SHOULDER STABILITY
FOREARM PUSH-UP**

Primary muscles:
Deltoids,
rotator cuff muscles,
triceps brachii

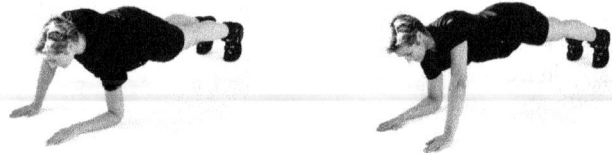

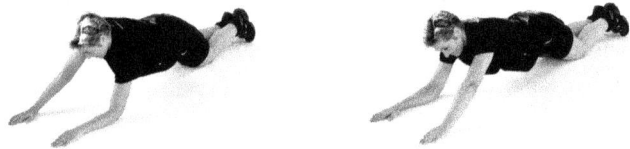

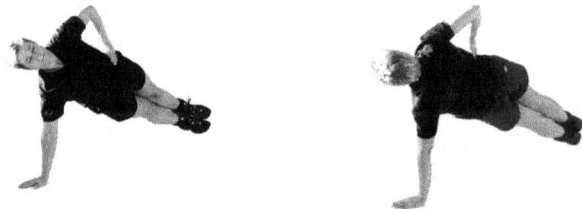

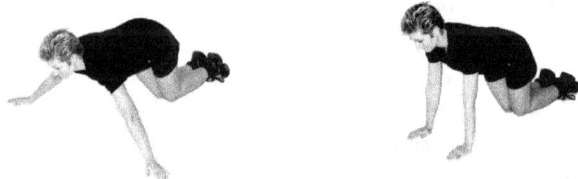

**SHOULDER STABILITY
DIAGONAL PLANK ON
FOREARM**

Primary muscles:
Deltoids, rotator cuff
muscles, triceps brachii

**SHOULDER STABILITY
TURNING SIDEPLANK**

Primary muscles:
Deltoids,
rotator cuff muscles,
triceps brachii

**SHOULDER STABILITY
ARM SLIDING**

Primary muscles:
Deltoids,
rotator cuff muscles,
triceps brachii

Plank position on hands and toes. Hands on the floor shoulder-width apart. Bend one elbow and lower the forearm down to the floor, then the other. Extend the elbow of the first arm, then the other. Repeat.	Contract the core muscles to stabilize the body. After a set with one arm leading, do a set with the other arm leading.	On knees or toes. Different shoulder angle.
Plank position on hands and lower legs. Hands on the floor shoulder-width apart. Arms diagonally in front of the body. Bend one elbow and lower one forearm to the floor, then the other forearm to the floor. Extend the first elbow, then the other to get bak up. Repeat.	Contract the core muscles to stabilize the body.	On knees or toes. Different angle at the shoulders.
Side plank position. One hand on the floor. Side of foot or feet on the floor. Free arm position is optional. Turn ¼ and put both hands on the floor (plank). Turn ¼, to the opposite side with the opposite hand supporting. Repeat back.	For intermediate exercises. For balance work. Contract the core muscles to stabilize the body.	On the hands or forearms.
Plank position. Hands and lower legs on the floor. Hands directly under the shoulders in a push-up position. Slide the arms out to the side. Adduct the arms back in.	For advanced exercisers Contract the core muscles to stabilize the body.	On knees or toes. Different angles.

EXERCISE	TECHNIQUES	

**SHOULDER STABILITY
PLANK POSITION
(WITH OR WITHOUT SLIDE)**

Primary muscles:
Deltoids, triceps brachii,
rotator cuff muscles

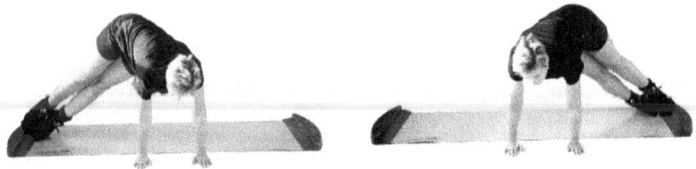

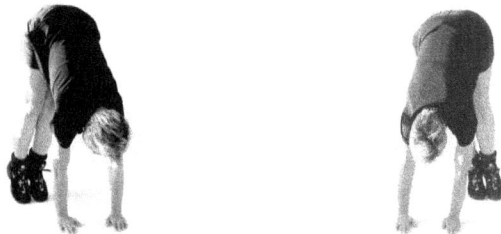

**SHOULDER STABILITY
WITH LATERAL TRAVELLING**

Primary muscles:
Deltoids, triceps brachii,
rotator cuff muscles

**SHOULDER, DYNAMIC
ONE-ARM STABILIZATION
SIDE PLANK POSITION**

Primary muscles:
Deltoids, triceps brachii,
rotator cuff muscles,
obliques, rectus abdominis

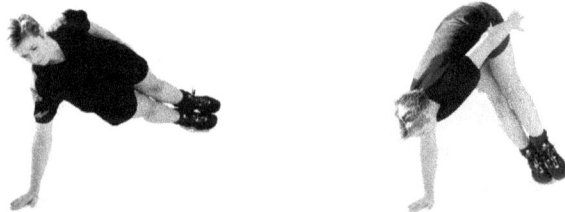

**SHOULDER, ISOMETRIC
ONE-ARM STABILIZATION
SIDE PLANK POSITION**

Primary muscles:
Deltoids,
rotator cuff muscles

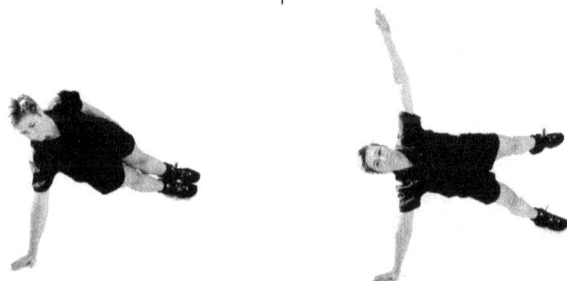

Standing on a slide board. Feet together. Torso forward. Hands on the floor. Bodyweight on the arms. Let the legs slide to one side. Contract your abs and pull the legs to the other side.	Contract the core muscles to stabilize the body. A certain amount of hamstring flexibility is required.	Small or large range of motion.
Standing. Feet together. Torso forward. Hands on the floor. Bodyweight on the arms. Swing the legs sideways to a new position. Lift the hands and move them to the legs. Swing the legs sideways again (maybe back). Lift both hands and move them to the legs	Contract the core muscles to stabilize the body. A certain amount of hamstring flexibility is required.	Small or large range of motion.
Side plank position. One hand on the floor, the other at the side of the torso. Contract the abdominals and pull legs sidewards closer to the hand. Let the legs slide back.	For advanced exercisers. Contract the core muscles to stabilize the body.	Dynamic or isometric exercise.
Side plank position. One hand on the floor, the other at the side of the torso. Support on one or both feet. Lower and lift the body, down and up laterally, frontal plane. Or hold position. Lift the top leg for extra work.	For advanced exercisers. Contract the core muscles to stabilize the body.	Dynamic or isometric exercise.

4 | Chest Exercises

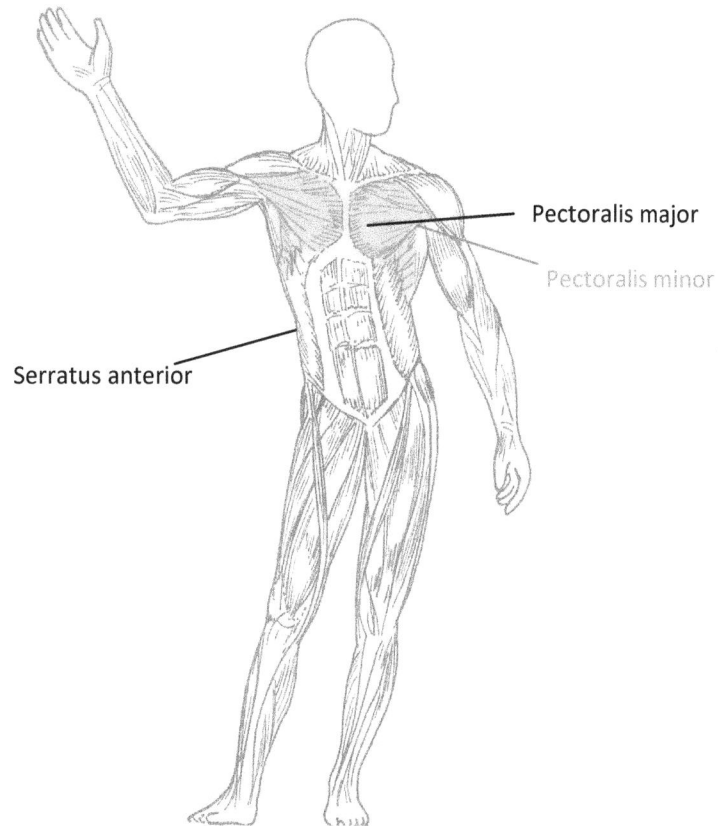

Pectoralis major

Pectoralis minor

Serratus anterior

CROSS OVER

Primary muscles:
Pectoralis major,
anterior deltoid

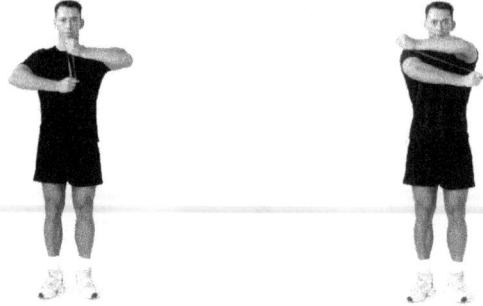

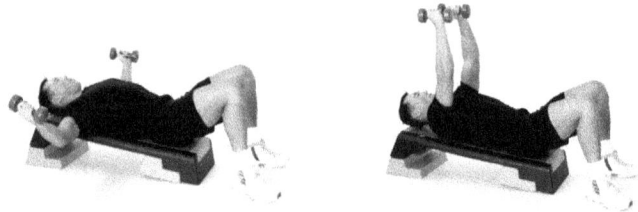

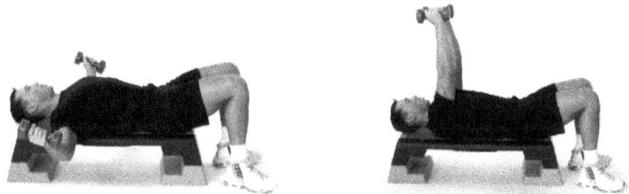

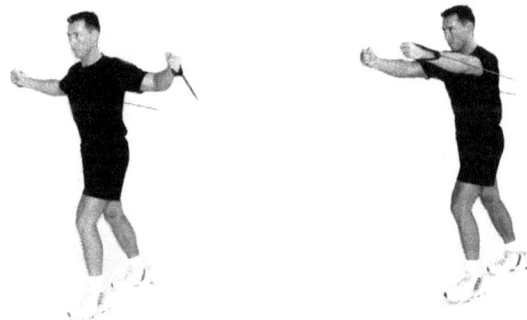

INCLINE CHEST FLYS

Primary muscles:
Pectoralis major,
anterior deltoid

**CHEST FLYS
(DUMBBELL FLYS)**

Primary muscles:
Pectoralis major,
anterior deltoid

**CHEST FLYS, STANDING
WITH RESISTANCE BAND
OR TUBE**

Primary muscles:
Pectoralis major,
anterior deltoid

Standing. Hold rubberband. The band is vertical. One hand at the top end, other hand at the bottom. The shoulders are lowered. Press the arms past each other, a chest crossover, so the rubberband is stretched. Return with control.	Limited range of motion. Limited functionality. Some toning effect. Keep shoulder blades in place, so the movement comes from the chest muscles working (contraction), not the shoulders sliding forward. After a set, repeat with the other arm at the top	Different body/leg position.
Supine on an incline bench. Arms slightly bent and out to the side in horizontal plane. Hold the dumbbells with the palms facing upwards. Lift, adduct, the arms and bring them close together over the chest, stop just before vertical. Avoid movement of elbows. Return to starting position.	Stop downward movement, when the hands are at the same height as the shoulders – do not lower the arms too much with heavy dumbbells – in order not to overload the shoulder ligaments. Stop arms around or before vertical – with gravity still pulling at the dumbbells.	Different arm/leg position. One or both arms. On bench or ball.
Supine on a flat bench. The arms slightly bent and to the side in horizontal plane. Hold the dumbbells in the hands, palms face upwards. Lift, adduct, the arms and bring them close together over the chest, stop just before vertical. Avoid movement of elbows. Return to starting position.	Chest isolation exercise. Works the pectoralis (and shoulder), not the triceps. In the end range of motion the chest muscles are in their weakest position; Exercise caution, especially with heavy weights. Stop downward movement, when the arms are at shoulder level.	Different arm/leg position. Different body position, incline or decline. One or both arms. A bodybar in one hand. On floor, bench or ball.
Standing. Tube anchored behind (or to the side of) the body and held by the hands. Arms slightly bent and to the side in horizontal plane. Adduct the arms, pull them in front of the chest. Return to starting position.	Standing flys are more functional than supine flys – you are erect and must stabilize your body. Stop outward movement, when the arms are in line with the body – not too for back with heavy resistance – to avoid overloading the shoulders.	Different arm/body/leg position. Different angle between the arms and the body.

EXERCISE	TECHNIQUE

PULLOVER

Primary muscles:
Pectoralis major,
serratus anterior,
latissimus dorsi

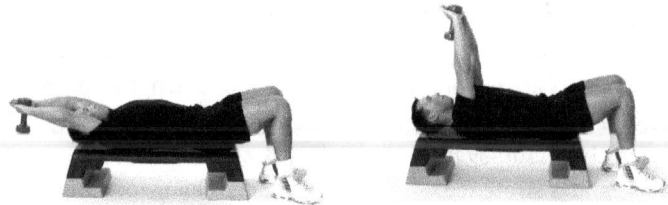

CHEST PRESS, STANDING

Primary muscles:
Pectoralis major and minor,
triceps brachiii,
anterior deltoid

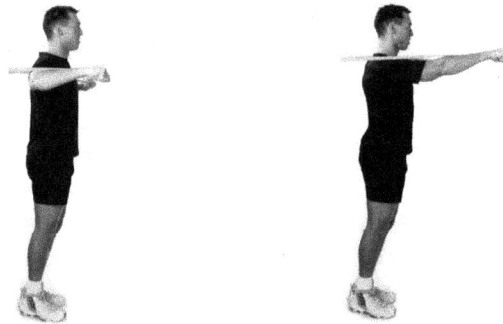

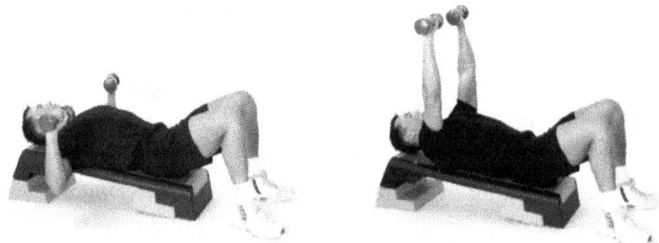

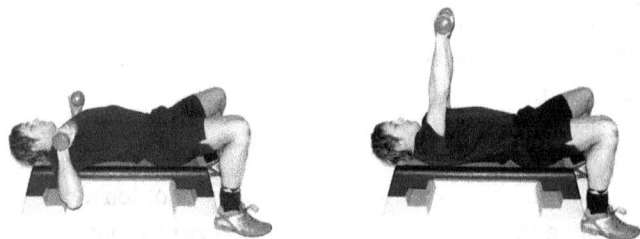

**INCLINE DUMBBELL
(CHEST) PRESS**

Primary muscles:
Pectoralis major and minor,
triceps brachiii,
anterior deltoid

**CHEST PRESS
(SUPINE DUMBBELL PRESS)**

Primary muscles:
Pectoralis major and minor,
triceps brachii,
anterior deltoid

TECHNIQUE	DETAIL	VARIATION
Supine. The arms in vertical position. Hold dumbbell or barbell. Lower the arms behind the head. The movement stops, when the upper arms are close to the ears. Lift/pull the arms back up to vertical. No elbow movement throughout the movement.	With a dumbbell use the 'triangle'-grip. Thumbs and indexfingers around the dumbbell and in contact with each other, slide them over each other to form a 'lock'. Stop upward movement just before vertical, with gravity still pulling on the dumbbell.	Different arm/body/leg position. Lie across the bench, so the lower back is free, unsupported, and the neck supported. With barbell or dumbbell(s). Tube/band from behind the body for a larger ROM working against resistance.
Standing. Band/tube anchored behind (or to the side of) the body. Arms bent, elbows out and back in the horizontal plane. Band/tube ends in the hands. Press the arms forward to a position together in front of the body. Return back to the starting position.	Standing press exercises are more functional than supine exercises. A staggered foot position gives better balance and is more sports specific.	Different body/leg position. One or both arms. Different grip: Pronated, neutral grip (mid-pronated), with rotation. With tube or band.
Supine on an incline bench. Arms bent and out, 80-90 degree angle to the torso. Hold dumbbells in hands. The hands close to the shoulders, forearms perpendicular to the floor. Press the arms vertically upwards and stop above the chest. Lower arms back down.	Stop downward movement, when the arms are in line with the body – do not lower too far, especially not with heavy dumbbells – do not overload the shoulder ligaments.	Different body/leg position. One or both arms. Different grip: Pronated, neutral grip (mid-pronated), with rotation. With tube or band.
Supine on a flat bench. Arms bent and out, 80-90 degree angle to the torso. Hold dumbbells in hands. The hands close to the shoulders, forearms perpendicular to floor. Press the arms vertically upwards and stop over the chest. Lower arms back down.	Stop downward movement, when the arms are in line with the body – do not lower too far, especially not with heavy dumbbells – do not overload the shoulder ligaments.	Different body/leg position. One or both arms. Different grip: Pronated, neutral grip (mid-pronated), with rotation. With tube or band.

EXERCISE	TECHNIQUE

**CHEST PRESS
WITH ROTATION
(DUMBBELL PRESS WITH
ROTATION)**

Primary muscles:
Pectoralis major and minor,
triceps brachii, anterior deltoid

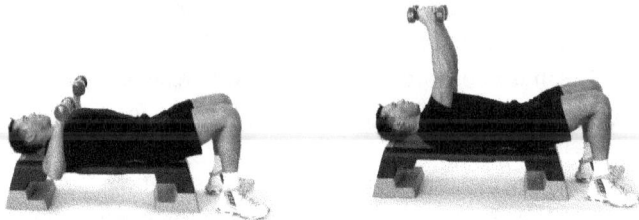

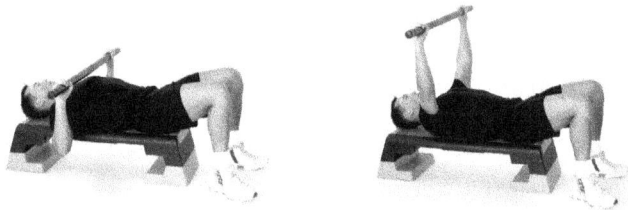

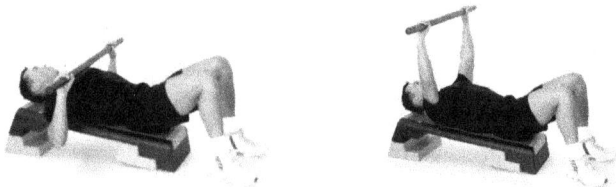

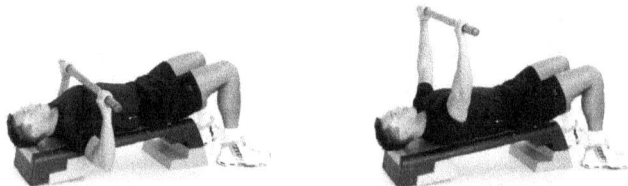

**BENCH PRESS
(SUPINE BARBELL PRESS)**

Primary muscles:
Pectoralis major,
triceps brachii,
anterior deltoid

INCLINE BARBELL PRESS

Primary muscles:
Pectoralis major,
triceps brachii,
anterior deltoid

DECLINE BARBELL PRESS

Primary muscles:
Pectoralis major,
triceps brachii,
anterior deltoid

TECHNIQUE	ADVICE	VARIATION
Supine. Arms bent and at a 80-90 degr. angle to the torso. Hold dumbbells in the hands. Hands close to shoulders. Palms forward. Press the arms upwards and rotate the arms, bringing the hands close together in top position. Lower back down with control.	A preferred chest exercise; large range of motion with limited risk of overloading the elbows and shoulders.	Different body/leg position. One or both arms.
Supine. Arms bent and at a 80-90 degree angle to the torso. Wide grip on barbell. Wrists are in neutral position. Press the arms upwards without locking the elbows. Barbell right above forearm. Barbell is lowered to the middle of the chest.	Tip: Stop just before touching the chest in order to keep the tension and to avoid using the chest as a trampoline. Options: Narrow grip (triceps focus) or wide grip (chest focus).	**FLOOR BARBELL PRESS** Supine on floor, thereby limiting range of motion; focus on the 'top' of the exercise. **GUILLOTINE** Barbell is lowered towards the neck. For advanced exercisers, requires attention and control.
Supine. Bench 30-60 degree incline. Position head at the high end. Wide grip on barbell, overhand grip. Press the arms up without locking the elbows. When upper arms are horizontal, the forearms are perpendicular to them (90 degree elbow angle). Lower barbell to chest, collarbone, with control.	The wrists in neutral position. Do not let the wrists bend back- or forwards with barbell. Tip: Stop just before touching the chest in order to keep the tension and to avoid using the chest as a trampoline.	With barbell or dumbbells. With dumbbells: With different grip: Neutral, pronated, with rotation.
Supine. Bench 30-60 degree decline. Head at the low end. Wide grip on barbell, overhand grip. Press the arms up without locking the elbows. When the upper arms are at horizontal, forearms are perpendicular to them. Lower barbell to chest.	The wrists in neutral position. Do not let the wrists bend back- or forward with barbell. Positions with the head down may feel uncomfortable. Should be limited to shorter periods at a time. Not for beginners, the elderly or deconditioned target groups.	With barbell or dumbbells. With dumbbells: With different grip: Neutral, pronated, with rotation.

EXERCISE	TECHNIQUE	
CHEST SQUEEZE ISOMETRICALLY Primary muscles: Pectoralis major, triceps brachii		
PUSH-UP, WIDE (CHEST PUSH-UP) Primary muscles: Pectoralis major, triceps brachii, anterior deltoid		
PUSH-UP, SUPER WIDE Primary muscles: Pectoralis major, triceps brachii, anterior deltoid		
HINDU PUSH-UP Primary muscles: Pectoralis major, triceps brachii, anterior deltoid		

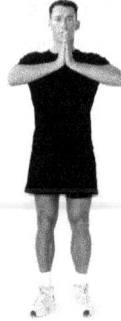

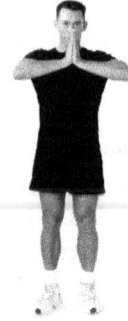

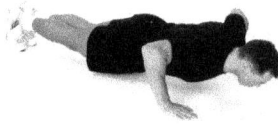

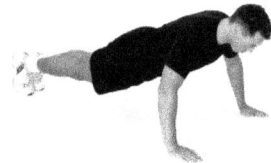

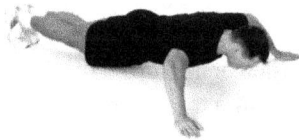

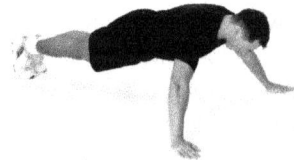

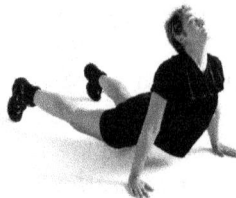

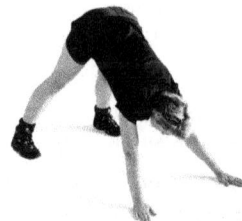

Standing. The arms in horizontal plane. The palms press against each other in front of the chest. The arms press as hard as possible. Keep contracting and hold for 5-7 seconds or more. Relax and repeat.	Limited functionality. Slight toning effect. Remember to keep breathing. Remember to relax the neck and shoulders as much as possible and focus on the chest.	Different body/leg position. Standing, kneeling, sitting. **CHEST SQUEEZE WITH LIFT** The arms bent 90 degrees and forearms together in front of the body. Lift the arms up and down in front of the body.
Plank position. Toes on floor. Hands on the floor, shoulder-width or more apart. When upper arms are horizontal, forearms are perpendicular to them. Extend the arms without locking the elbows. Bend the arms and lower the body, stop approx. 4 inches, 10 cm, before chest touches the floor.	Contract the core muscles to stabilize the body. Neck in neutral position. Shoulder blades are held in neutral position. Avoid locking the elbows in top position.	Different body/leg position. With weight plate on the back. **TRAVELLING PUSH-UP** The body moves sideways, back and forth, or continues to the side
Plank position. Toes on the floor. Hands on the floor, super wide. Hands slightly outwards. Extend the arms without locking the elbows. Bend the arms and lower the body, stop approx. 4 inches, 10 cm, before the chest touches the floor.	Contract the core muscles to stabilize the body. Neck in neutral position. Shoulder blades are held in neutral position. Avoid locking the elbows in top position.	Different body/leg position. - Against a wall, or feet or arms on top of a bench. With weight plate on the back.
Plank position. Hands wider than shoulder-width apart. Push the buttocks backwards into yoga 'downward dog'. Lift the heels and bend the arms and lower the head/torso down between the arms in a circular movement. End in a yoga 'dog' with the head op. Push back into pike position.	For advanced exercisers. Super push-up exercise, which strengthens and stretches several muscles and massage the organs, when bending and extending the body. Avoid locking the elbows in top position.	Different body/leg position. **DIVE BOMBER** As a hindu push-up, but more arm/chest/shoulder strength work; push back with a circular movement; down and up in the same way. This version has less focus on flexibility than the hindu push-up.

EXERCISE	TECHNIQUE

PUSH JACK

Primary muscles:
Pectoralis major,
triceps brachii,
anterior deltoid

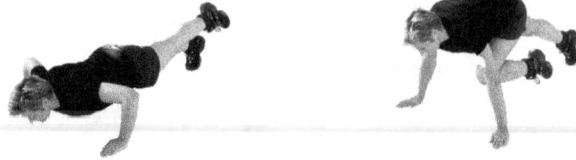

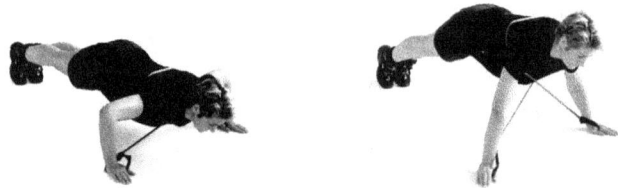

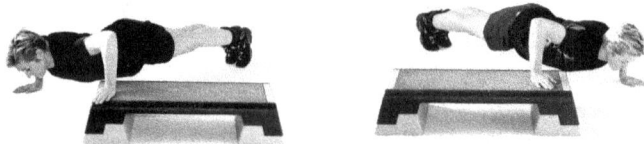

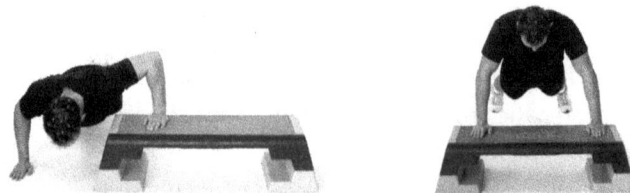

PUSH-UP
WITH BAND OR TUBE

Primary muscles:
Pectoralis major,
triceps brachii,
anterior deltoid

PUSH-UP, DIAGONAL
ON BENCH

Primary muscles:
Pectoralis major,
triceps brachii,
anterior deltoid

PUSH-UP, TRAVELLING,
ON BENCH

Primary muscles:
Pectoralis major,
triceps brachii,
anterior deltoid

Plank position. Toes on the floor. Hands on the floor, wider than shoulder-width apart. Arms push-up without locking elbows, at the same time pull one leg up towards the body. Arms bend, lower the body, and return the leg to the starting position. Repeat and change leg.	Contract the core muscles to stabilize the body. Neck in neutral position. Avoid locking elbows in the top position.	Different body/leg position. Feet on floor, bench or ball.
Plank position. On toes. Hands on the floor, shoulder-width apart. Tube or band around the back (chest level) crossed in front of the chest and under the hands. Extend the arms, without locking the elbows. Bend the arms bend and lower the body. Stop 4 inches, 10 cm, before chest touches the floor.	Contract the core muscles to stabilize the body. Neck in neutral position. Shoulder blades in neutral position. Avoid locking elbows in the top position.	Standing, kneeling, supporting on a wall.
Plank position. Toes on the floor. One hand on the bench, the other hand on the floor. Arms wide. Push-up without locking the elbows. Bend the arms and lower the body. Stop approx. 4 inches, 10 cm, before the chest touches the floor. Push-up. Change side.	Contract the core muscles to stabilize the body. Neck in neutral position. Shoulder blades in neutral position. Avoid locking elbows in the top position.	You can change arm and side with an explosive push up, or you can do a series of push-ups changing side on the way. Bench can be turned (aligned with the body)
Plank position. The hands wide on the bench, arms bent. 1) Arms push-up and land side by side at one end of the bench. 2) One hand on the floor and lower the body. 3) Push back up on the bench, hands shoulder-width apart. 4) Hands out wide, one on the floor, lower down. Push-up.	Contract the core muscles to stabilize the body. Neck in neutral position. Shoulder blades in neutral position. Avoid locking elbows in the top position in all of the different positions.	Different leg position.

EXERCISE	TECHNIQUE

PUSH-UP, INCLINE

Primary muscles:
Pectoralis major,
triceps brachii,
anterior deltoid

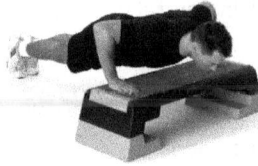

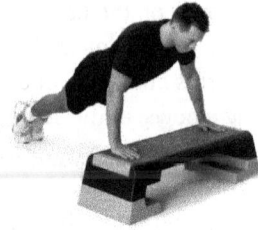

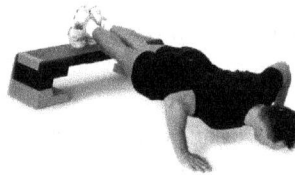

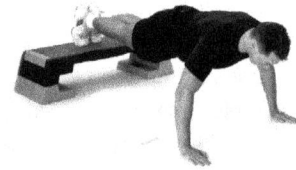

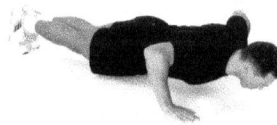

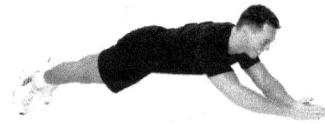

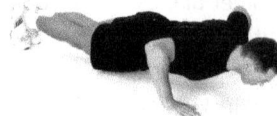

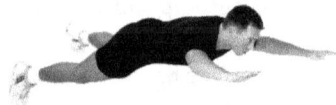

PUSH-UP, DECLINE

Primary muscles:
Pectoralis major,
triceps brachii,
anterior deltoid

PUSH-UP WITH CLAP

Primary muscles:
Pectoralis major,
triceps brachii,
anterior deltoid

EXPLOSIVE PUSH-UP

Primary muscles:
Pectoralis major,
triceps brachii,
anterior deltoid

Plank position. Toes on the floor. Hands, wider than shoulder-width apart on bench, incline body position. The arms push-up, extend completely without locking the elbows. Bend the arms and lower the body. Stop approx. 4 inches, 10 cm, before the chest touches the floor.	The incline position, shorter lever arm, makes the exercise easier. Contract the core muscles to stabilize the body. Neck and shoulder blades in neutral position. Avoid locking elbows in top position.	Standing, kneeling, supporting on a wall. Different body angle. **MEDICINE BALL PUSH-UP** With both feet on a medicine ball and each hand on a medicine ball (can also be performed on other stability equipment).
Plank position. Feet/legs on a bench. The hands on the floor, wider than shoulder-width apart. Body in decline position. The arms push-up, extend completely without locking the elbows. Bend the arms and lower the body. Stop approx. 4 inches, 10 cm, before the chest touches the floor.	For advanced exercisers. The decline position is a little harder (focus on shoulders). Note: Positions with the head down may feel uncomfortable. Limit to shorter periods of time. Not for beginners, the elderly or the deconditioned. Contract the core muscles to stabilize the body.	Leg/feet rest on a ball, bench or similar. Different body angle. Legs straight or bent, together or apart.
Plank position. Toes on the floor. Hands on the floor shoulder-width apart. Arms push-up explosively, so the body is airborne. Then clap the hands. When landing bend the arms, to break the fall and lower the body. Stop approx. 4 inches, 10 cm, before the chest touches the floor.	For advanced exercisers. Hard on the wrists. Contract the core muscles to stabilize the body.	Different leg position
Plank position. Toes on the floor. Hands on the floor, shoulder-width or wider. Extend the arms explosively, so the whole body is propelled into the air. When landing the arms break the fall, so the body is lowered with control. Stop appox. 4 inches, 10 cm, before chest touches the floor.	For very advances exercisers. Hard on the wrists. Contract the core muscles to stabilize the body. Contract the thighs to protect the knees. Avoid landing with legs too wide (hard on knees).	Different leg position. One leg may be flexed, so the leg helps to push the body off the ground. On the spot or with forward travelling.

TRAVELLING PUSH-UP

Primary muscles:
Pectoralis major,
triceps brachii, deltoids,
transversus abdominis

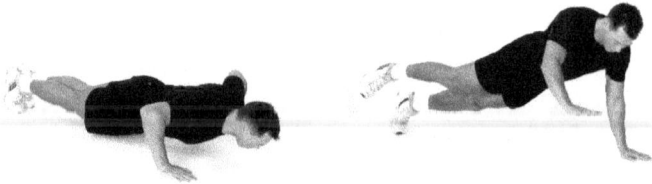

FREE FALL, WIDE

Primary muscles:
Pectoralis major,
triceps brachii,
anterior deltoid

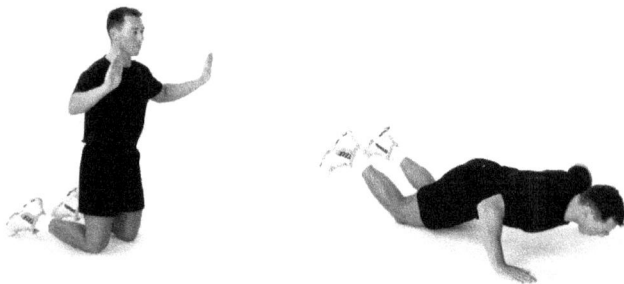

SERRATUS PUSH SUPINE

Primary muscles:
Serratus anterior,
pectoralis major

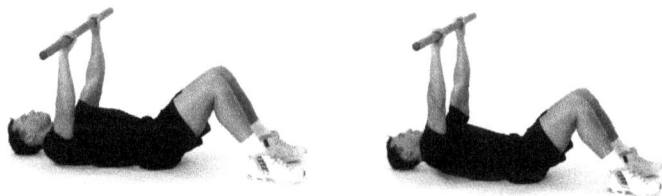

SERRATUS PLANK PRESS

Primary muscles:
Serratus anterior,
pectoralis major,
transversus abdominis

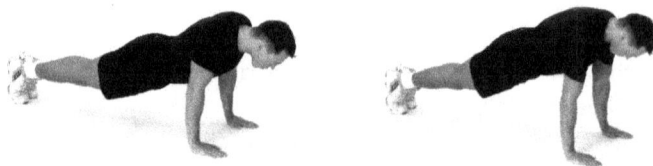

Plank position. Toes on the floor. Hands on the floor, shoulder-width, or wider apart. The arms push up, extend, without locking the elbows. At the same time the arms extend, one arm is moved to the side. Lower and push-up again. Repeat	Contract the core muscles to stabilize the body. Neck in neutral position. Shoulder blades in neutral position.	Feet either remain in the same place, or the legs take a step, when the arms move out. On floor or bench. **PUSH-UP CIRCLE** Advanced exercise: Push-up with power, the body moves to the side. Continue in a circle. Feet remain in the same place.
Kneeling. Arms bent and at horizontal plane. The body falls forward and the arms break the fall gently. Push up, extend the arms forcefully, so the body is pushed back to standing position.	For advanced exercisers. Standing version requires years of basic training for the wrists. Especially if performed on a hardwood floor. Start with a small range of motion and a landing mat. Contract the core muscles to stabilize the body.	Different body/leg position On the feet or the knees. Landing on a bench, mat, BOSU or floor.
Supine. Barbell in hands. Arms vertical and shoulder-width apart. Contract the chest muscles and 'push' the bodybar up and down with straight arms – a shoulder blade movement, protraction. Lower with control.	Lying down on the muscles, you are working, is not the optimal workout position.	Different leg position. On bench or ball.
Plank position. On the hands and knees or toes. The arms are straight, and there is no movement in the elbow joint. Chest and core muscles contract. Abduct, protract, the shoulder blades. Return with control.	Contract the core muscles to stabilize the body. Important stability exercise for the torso.	Different leg position. The hands on floor, bench or ball.

5 | Back Exercises

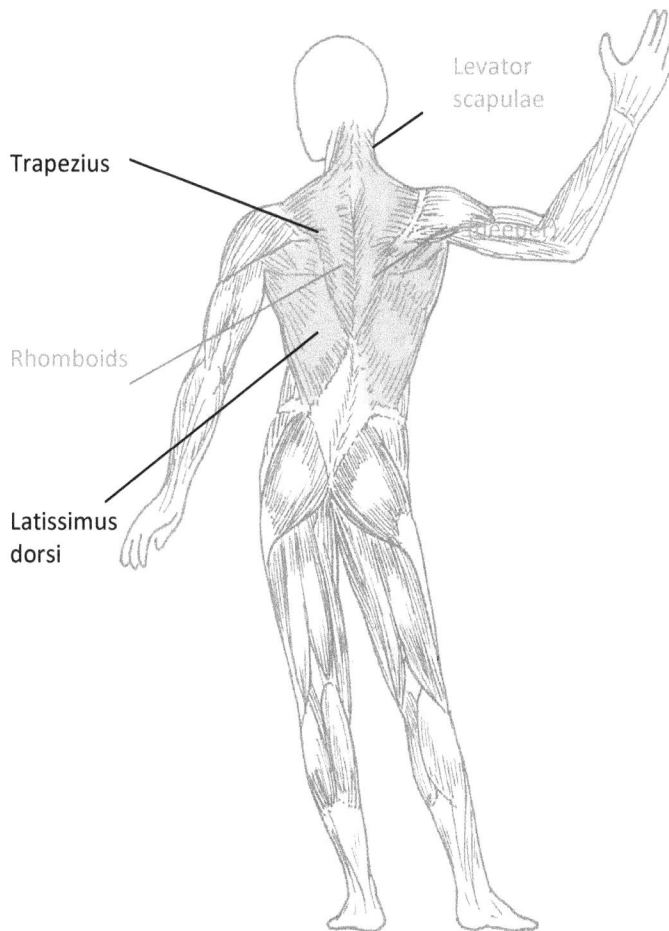

Levator
scapulae

Trapezius

Rhomboids

Latissimus
dorsi

EXERCISE	TECHNIQUE	
UNILATERAL STABILITY SHRUG Primary muscles: Trapezius, levator scapulae		
SHRUGS Primary muscles: Trapezius, levator scapulae		
SHRUGS WITH CIRCLES Primary muscles: Trapezius, levator scapulae		
POWER SHRUGS (JUMP SHRUG) Primary muscles: Trapezius, levator scapulae		

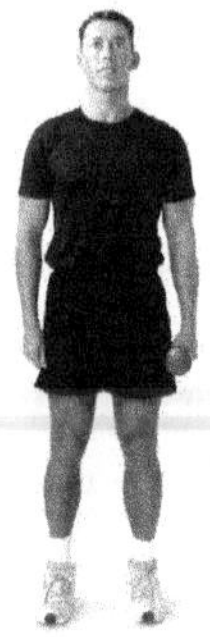

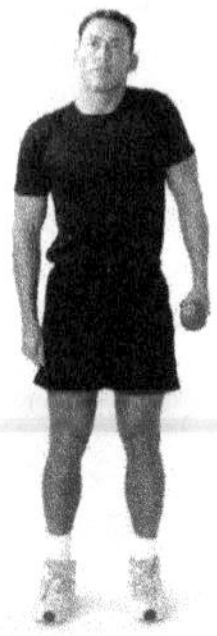

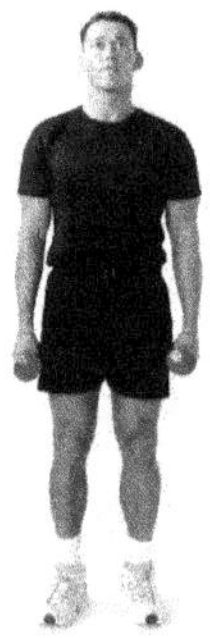

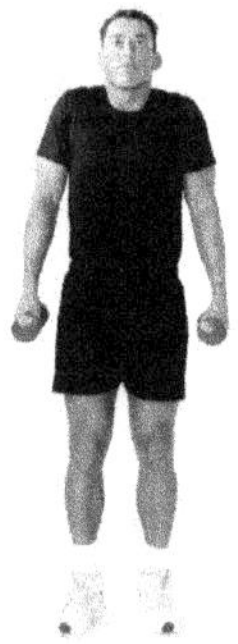

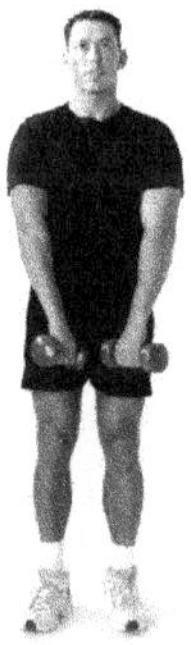

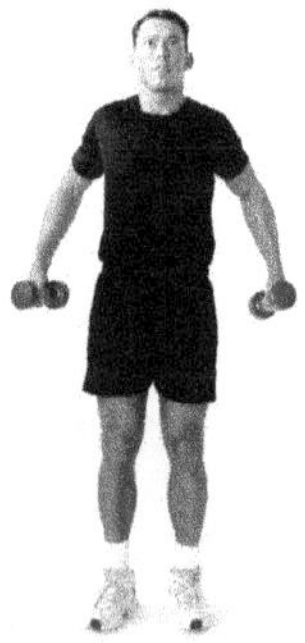

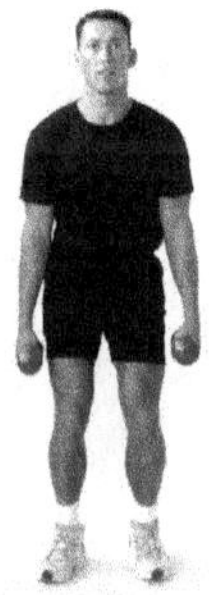

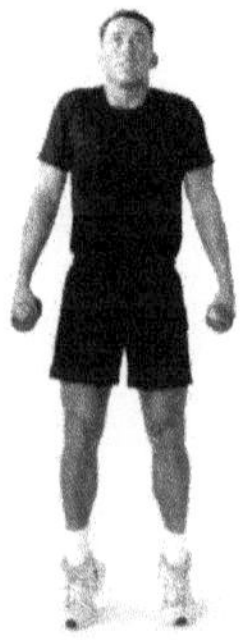

Standing. Feet shoulder-width apart, legs slightly bent. Arms at sides, shoulder blades in neutral. Heavy dumbbell in one hand. Lift the shoulder towards the ear. Lift straight up in the frontal plane – avoid pulling the shoulder forward. Lower.	Stand in front or mirror. Check that the body appears 'symmetrical', shoulders level. Avoid sidebending, when you lift the dumbbell. Good exercise for releasing or preventing tension of the neck muscles and headaches. Provides core stability work.	With dumbbell(s), barbell, with tube or band.
Standing. Feet shoulder-width apart, legs slightly bent. Arms at sides, shoulder-blades in neutral. Lift the shoulders. Lift straight up in trontal plane – avoid pulling the shoulders forward. Lower with control.	One of the best exercises for strength training the neck and reducing tension in the neck area. Basic exercise for weightlifting exercises.	Different leg position. Unilateral, bilateral. With dumbbell(s), barbell (in front of or behind the body). With tube or band.
Standing. Feet shoulder-width apart. Arms at sides. Lift the shoulders, and at the same time circle the shoulders forward, upward, backward and down. A slow controlled movement.	The exercise does not provide additional effect compared to traditional shrugs – it does not provide increased strength work for the trapezius, but is used for variety. After a set, repeat circling the opposite way.	Different leg position. Unilateral, bilateral. With the dumbbell(s), barbell (in front of or behind the body), with tube or band.
Standing. Leg slightly bent and feet shoulder-width apart. Arms at side. Shoulder blades in neutral. One dumbbell in each hand. Bend the legs slightly and quickly and jump. When the legs extend explosively, lift the shoulders.	For advanced exercisers. Strength training for the shoulder girdle. Assistant exercise for weightlifting exercises. Requires a thorough warm-up.	Different leg position.

EXERCISE	TECHNIQUE

OVERHEAD PRESS SHRUG

Primary muscles:
Trapezius, levator scapulae

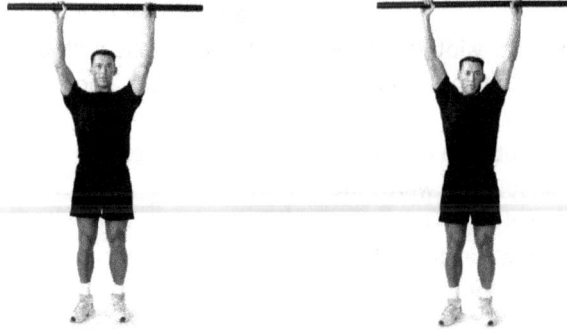

**BACK FLYS
(REVERSE FLYS)
ON ALL FOURS
WITH TUBE**

Primary muscles:
Rhomboids, middle trapezius,
posterior deltoid

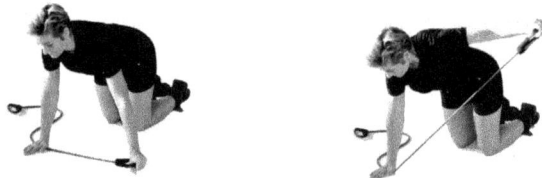

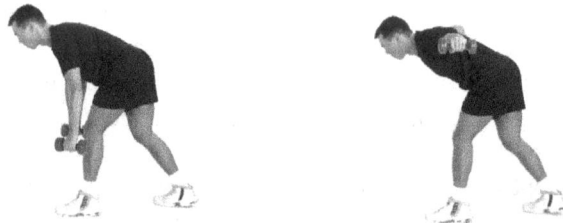

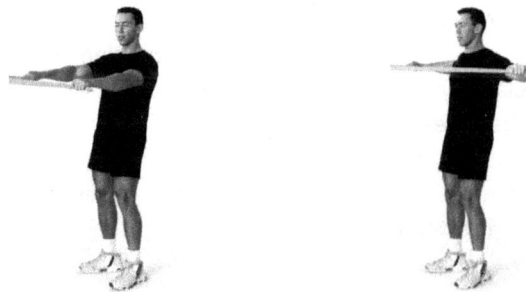

**BACK FLYS, BENT-OVER
(REVERSE FLYS)**

Primary muscles:
Rhomboids, middle trapezius,
posterior deltoid

**BACK FLYS, STANDING
(REVERSE FLYS)**

Primary muscles:
Rhomboids, middle trapezius,
posterior deltoid

TECHNIQUE	FOCUS	VARIATION
Standing. Feet shoulder-width apart. Legs slightly bent, ab muscles contracted. Wide overhand grip on barbell, both arms are held straight up as in shoulder press top position. Lift the shoulders. Lower with control.	Strength exercise for the shoulders. Small range of motion. Assistant exercise for weight-lifting exercises.	Special barbell with 'eyes'. With dumbbells.
On all fours. One hand holds one end of a tube. The other hand holds the handle. There must be some tension in the tube (no slack). Lift arm out and upwards. Focus on the muscles between the shoulder blades and not the arm. Return with control.	Contract the core muscles to stabilize the body. Elbow is slightly flexed, and in the same position throughout the movement. Lead the movement with the elbow.	With band or tube.
Standing (or sitting) with the back straight and forward. Dumbbells in hands. Arms down and slightly bent. Lift the arms out and up. Focus on the muscles between the shoulder blades, not the arms. Lower with control.	Contract the core muscles to stabilize the body. Elbow is slightly flexed, and in the same position throughout the movement. Lead the movement with the elbows.	Different leg position. Standing, sitting or prone on an Incline bench. Unilateral, bilateral. With dumbbell(s) or with tube or band.
Standing. Arms slightly bent and to the side in the horizontal plane. The hands hold the band/tube, which is anchored in front of the body. Pull arms backward, at chest level. Elbows lead. Focus on the back muscles between the shoulder blades, not the arms.	Contract the core muscles to stabilize the body. Elbow is slightly flexed, and in the same position throughout the movement. Lead the movement with the elbows.	Different leg position. Standing, sitting, kneeling. Unilateral, bilateral. The arms at different angles: **HIGH PULL** **LOW PULL** With tube or band.

EXERCISE	TECHNIQUE

**ARM PULL
(REVERSE)
PRONE**

Primary muscles:
Posterior deltoid,
trapezius, rhomboids

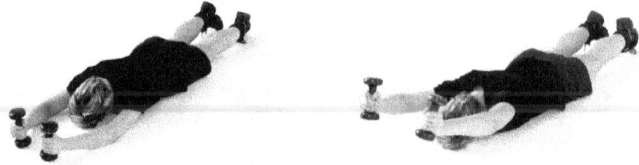

**BACK FLYS
(REVERSE FLYS)
DIAGONALLY UP
PRONE ON BENCH**

Primary muscles:
Rhomboids, middle trapezius,
posterior deltoid

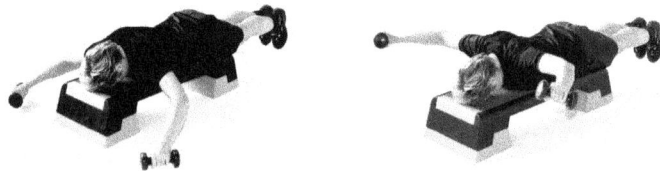

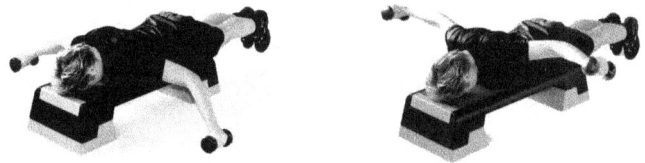

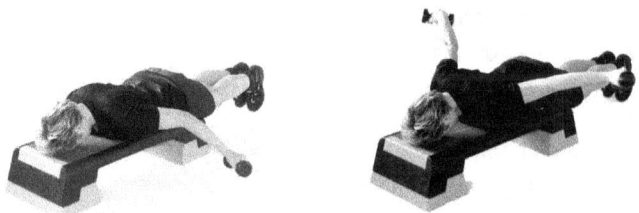

**BACK FLYS
(REVERSE FLYS)
PRONE ON BENCH**

Primary muscles:
Rhomboids, middle trapezius,
posterior deltoid

**BACK FLYS
(REVERSE FLYS)
DIAGONALLY DOWN
PRONE ON BENCH**

Primary muscles:
Rhomboids, middle trapezius,
Posterior deltoid

Prone. Arms extended up/forward. Upper arms by the side of the head. Palms face the floor or each other, neutral grip. The head is kept down. Lift the arms – with or without dumbbells in the hands. Lower with control.	Because of the prone position on the floor, range of motion is limited. Use as a variation. Keep the neck in neutral position.	Different arm/leg position. On bench, ball or floor. The arms can lift in different angles; the arms forward, diagonally forward, to the side, diagonally backward or back, close to the body.
Prone on bench. Arms diagonally upwards and outwards with the palms downwards or towards each other. Lift the arms. Elbows lead. Keep elbows slightly bent throughout the movement. Focus on the muscles between shoulder blades, not the arms.	Exercise for the shoulder girdle and the upper back. Neck in neutral position.	Different arm/leg position. On bench, ball or floor. Prone on floor, bench or ball (best on bench or ball, as you have a larger range of motion).
Prone on bench. Arms to the side – 90 degree angle to the torso. Palms downwards or towards each other. Lift the arms. Elbows lead. Keep elbows slightly bent throughout the movement. Focus on the muscles between the shoulder blades, not the arms.	Super exercise for posture improvement and body awareness. Neck in neutral position. Can also be performed with the elbows flexed 90 degrees.	Different arm/leg position. On bench, ball or floor. Prone on floor, bench or ball (best on bench or ball, as you have a larger range of motion).
Prone on bench. Arms diagonally back and out with palms downwards or towards each other. Lift the arms. Elbows lead. Keep elbows slightly bent throughout the movement. Focus on the shoulders and muscles between the shoulder blades,	Exercise for the shoulder girdle and the muscles of the upper back. Neck in neutral position.	Different arm/leg position. On bench, ball or floor. Prone on floor, bench or ball (best on bench or ball, as you have a larger range of motion).

EXERCISE	TECHNIQUE

ROWING, WIDE STANDING

Primary muscles:
Rhomboids,
posterior deltoid,
biceps brachii

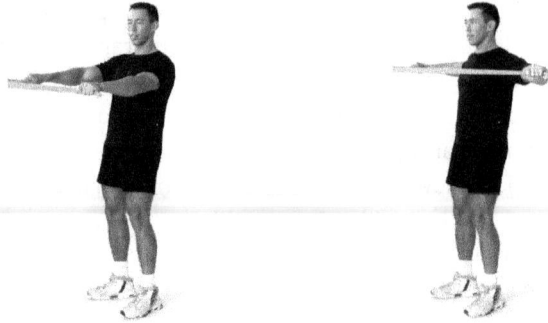

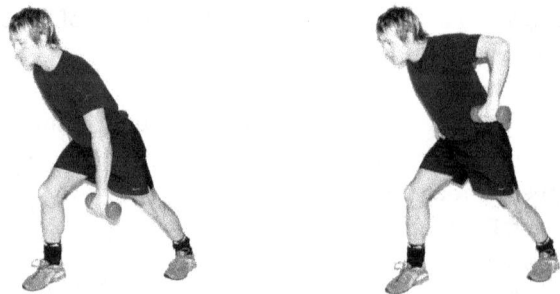

BENT-OVER ROWS ROWING, STANDING, FORWARD LEAN

Primary muscles:
Rhomboids, biceps
brachii, erector spinae,
posterior deltoid

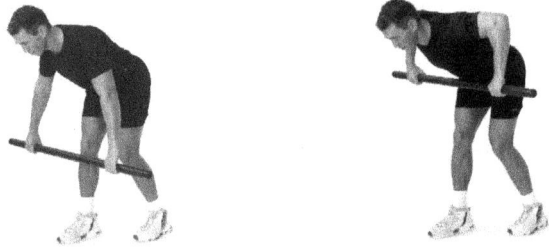

ONE-ARM ROWING, WIDE, KNEELING

Primary muscles:
Rhomboids,
latissimus dorsi, biceps brachii,
posterior deltoid

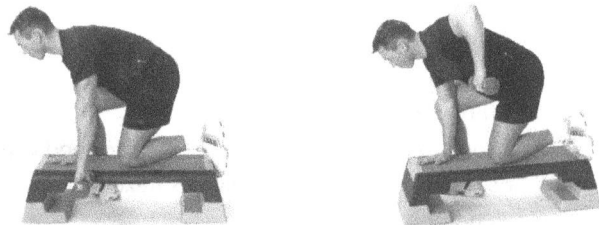

BENT-OVER ONE-ARM ROWS (ONE-ARM ROWING, STANDING, FORWARD LEAN

Primary muscles:
Rhomboids,
posterior deltoid,
biceps brachii

Standing. The arms slightly bent and to the side in horizontal plane The hands hold the tube. Pull towards the torso at chest level. Elbows lead. Focus on the back, muscles between the shoulder blades, not the arms.	Contract the core muscles to stabilize the body and keep the torso erect and stable.	Different body/leg position. One or both arms pull. Under-, over-, neutral grip. High pull, at neck level. With tube or band. With rubberband, unilaterallly, with rubberband in one hand.
Standing. Feet staggered. Arms slightly bent, straight down in front of the body. Hands overhand grip, wide, on barbell. Arms pull barbell upwards. Upper arms to the sides past horizontal. Forearms perpendicular (down). Focus on the muscles between shoulder blades. Lower.	With the torso supported or unsupported. When the body is unsupported, you work the lower back muscles isometrically. Alternatively you can rest the head or chest on a bench, wall bar or the like.	Different body/leg position. One or both arms pull. Under-, over-, neutral grip. **T-BAR ROWING** Standing, bent-over, feet wide apart straddling a barbell. Hold one end with both hands. Lift that end of the barbell to the torso. Lower with control.
Kneeling. One leg supporting on a (high) bench. Hand of the same side support on bench. Opposite foot on the floor. Free hand holds the dumbbell. Back is straight, core muscles contract. Shoulders and hips horizontal. Working arm vertical. Lift the arm up, retract the shoulder blade. Lower.	Contract the core muscles to stabilize the body, Keep the back straight. For isolation work: Avoid rotating the spine. Do not 'drop' the working arm without control. Keep the shoulders level.	With dumbbell or bodybar. **ROWING, RHOMBOIDS** Arm to the side, horizontal. Retract shoulder blades. **ROWING, LATISSIMUS DORSI** Arm close to the body, pull elbow past the ribs and well behind the body.
Standing. Forward lean. Feet staggered. Support hand on front leg. The working arm down. Lift the upper arm to the side above horizontal. Forearm vertically down. Elbow leads the movement, focus on the muscles between the shoulder blades. Lower with control.	The torso should not be too erect, because then you change the exercise. Recommended forward lean between 45-90 degrees.	Different body/legposition. Under-, over-, neutral grip. With dumbbell, tube or band.

EXERCISE	TECHNIQUE

SEATED ROWING, WIDE

Primary muscles:
Rhomboid, biceps
brachii, posterior deltoid,
erector spinae

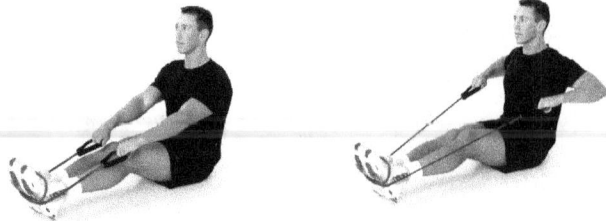

LAT PULLDOWN

Primary muscles:
Latissimus dorsi,
biceps brachii

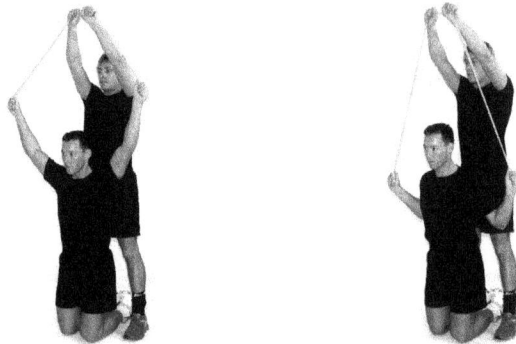

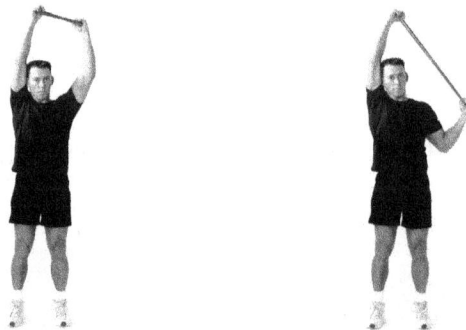

**UNILATERAL
LAT PULLDOWN**

Primary muscles:
Latissimus dorsi,
biceps brachii

PULL UP/CHIN UP

Primary muscles:
Latissimus dorsi, teres major,
biceps brachii, rhomboids

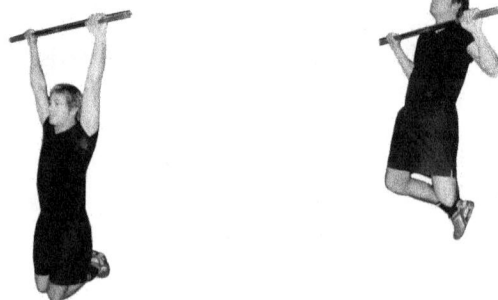

Sitting. Tube under feet. Arms forward, slightly bent. Pull the arms backwards just below chest level. Elbows lead. Focus on the back, muscles between the shoulder blades, not the arms. Return with control.	Contract the core muscles to stabilize the body. When moving the torso, the lower back, you involve the back extensors more – if so, do so in a controlled manner.	Different body/leg position. One or both arms pull. Under-, over-, neutral grip. **ROWING RHOMBOIDS** Arms to the side, horizontal plane. Adduct sholder blades **ROWING LATISSIMUS DORSI** Arms close to torso, pull the elbows close to the ribcage and well behind the body.
Kneeling (eg. with partner). Or standing (high). Tube/band held by partner or anchored at wall bar or door, well over the head. Hold the tube/band with a neutral or overhand grip. Lower the shoulders. Pull the arms down and into the side. Resist upward movement.	Lower the shoulders and shoulder blades before you pull down.	Different body position. Standing, kneeling, sitting, prone, supine. With tube or band.
Standing. Tube is held with the hand of the stationary arm, which is in vertical by the side of the head. Hold tube with opposite hand. Lower the shoulder. Pull working arm downwards in the frontal plane to the side of the torso. Return with control.	Start with the palms facing each other, neutral, to at avoid impingement of the shoulder. Stationary arm is kept as steady and stable as possible – in vertical or a little past.	Different body/leg position. Standing, kneeling, sitting, prone, supine. With rubberband, tube or band.
Hanging. Wide overhand grip. Lower the shoulders. Bend the arms. Pull the body up towards the bar. Lower with control.	You can make the exercise easier by supporting your feet on a bench, wall bar or partner. Wall bar: Pull the body up, so collarbone is level with hands. Chin-up bar: Lift the body, so the collarbone or neck touches the bar.	At wall bar use an over- or underhand grip. At the chin up bar use different grips and grip widths. **ONE-ARM CHIN UP** Grip bar with one hand, opposite hand grip around the wrist. Bend arm, lift the body. For advanced exercisers.

SEATED ROWING, NARROW (ROWING)

Primary muscles:
Latissimus dorsi,
biceps brachii,
posterior deltoid

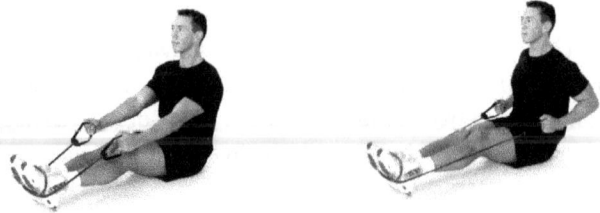

**PULLDOWN
(LAT PULLDOWN FRONT)
(STRAIGHT ARM PULLDOWN)**

Primary muscles:
Latissimus dorsi,
posterior deltoid

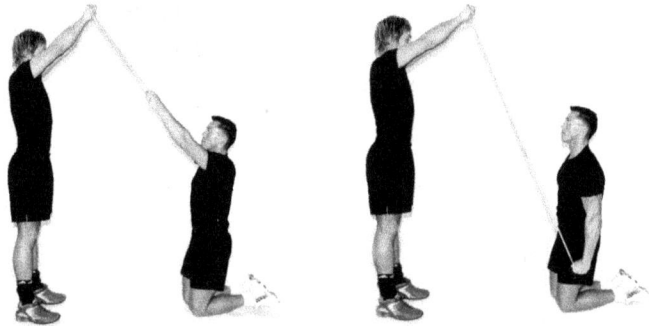

**PULLOVER
WITH RESISTANCE BAND**

Primary muscles:
Latissimus dorsi,
pectoralis major,
serratus anterior,
posterior deltoid

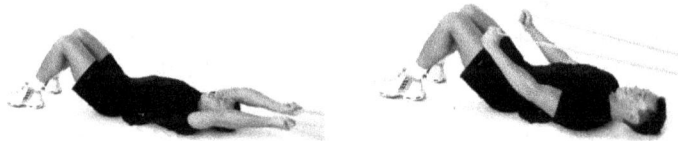

**SIDELYING OVERHEAD
PULLOVER**

Primary muscles:
Latissimus dorsi

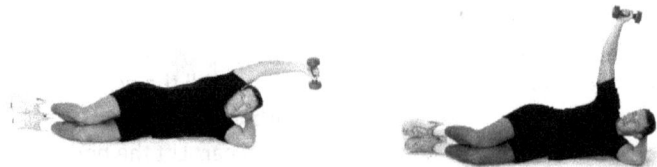

TECHNIQUE	NOTE	VARIATION
Sitting. Shoulders lowered. Arms straight forward in the sagittal plane. Pull arms towards the body, elbows pull back past the rib cage, sides of the torso. Focus on the back, not the arms. Return with control.	Contract the core muscles to stabilize the body. Keep the torso erect and immovable, if the exercise should target latissimus dorsi, Co-movement of the lower back involves back extensors. This must be with a controlled movement.	Different body/leg position. One or both arms pull. Under-, over- or neutral grip. With tube or band.
Kneeling or standing. Tube or band held by partner or a wall anchor well over the head. Tube/band ends in the hands. The arms are straight. Pull the tube downwards in front of the body, in the sagittal plane. Return with control.	Partner keeps the arms and tube steady and as high as possible for the best pull.	Different body position. Standing, kneeling, sitting. With tube or band.
Supine. Band anchored behind the body. Arms straight back, upper arms close to the ears. Pull the arms past the head and forward and down to the hips. Keep the arms straight throughout the movement. Return with control.	With a band you achieve a larger range of motion working against resistance – compared to free weights. With a dumbbell use 'triangle'-grip: Thumbs and indexfingers of both hands on the dumbbell touching each other. Slide over each other to form a 'lock'.	Different body/leg position. The arms straight or bent. You can lie across a bench with the lower back and the neck supported. With band, barbell or dumbbell.
Sidelying. A dumbbell in the top hand. Top, working, arm is in vertical. Lower the arm sideways down over the head. Raise the arm back up, close to vertical. Do not go past vertical as the exercise will change.	Contract the core muscles to stabilize the body. Stop upward movement just before vertical, to keep working against gravity. Limited range of motion with resistance (pull of gravity).	Sidelying on floor, bench or ball.

6 | Arm Exercises

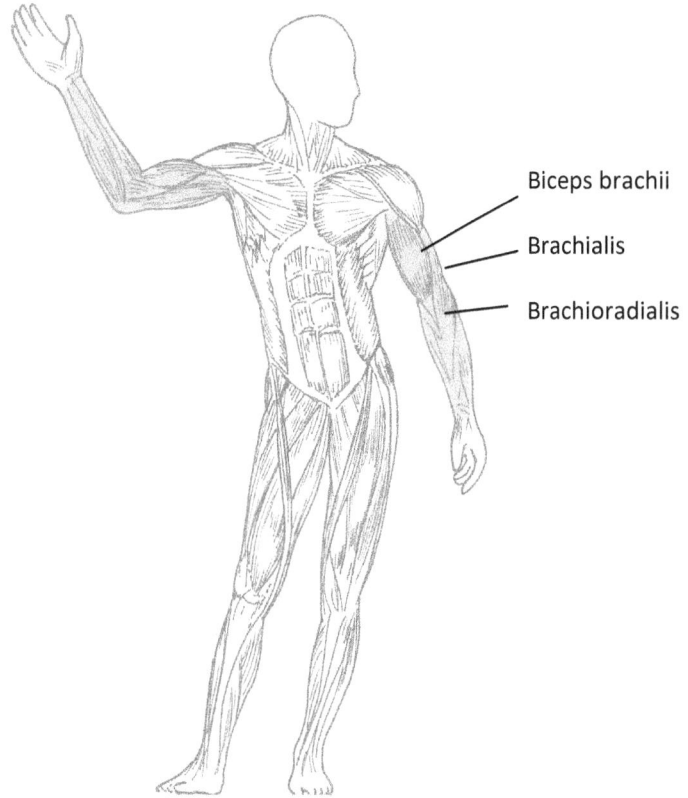

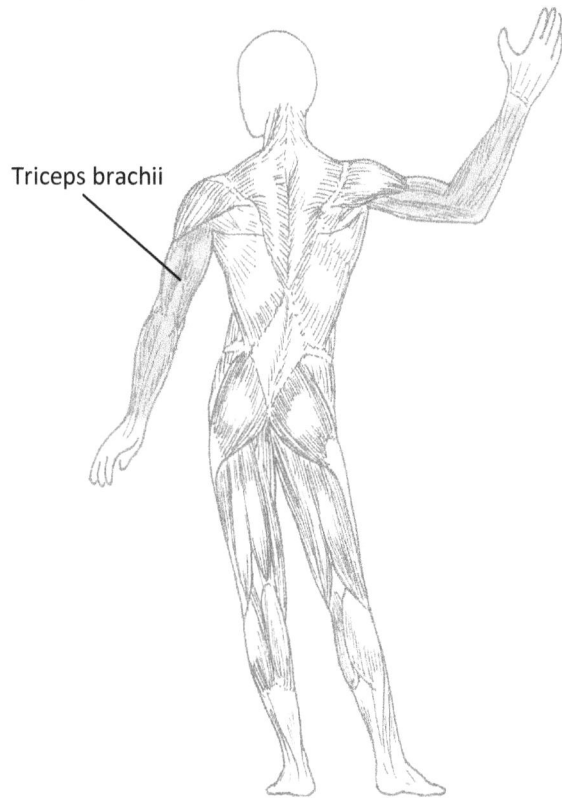

Biceps brachii

Brachialis

Brachioradialis

Triceps brachii

BICEPS BARBELL CURL

Primary muscles:
Biceps brachii, brachialis,
brachioradialis

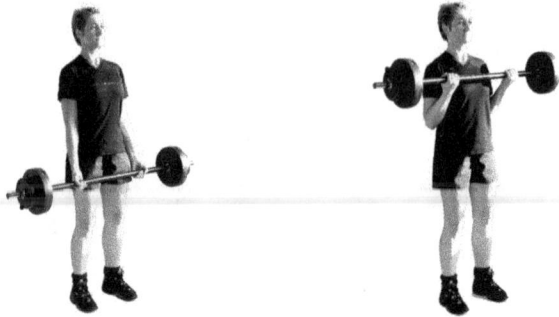

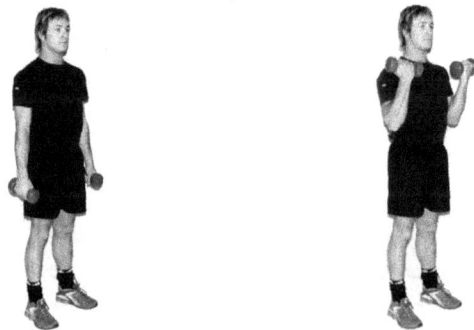

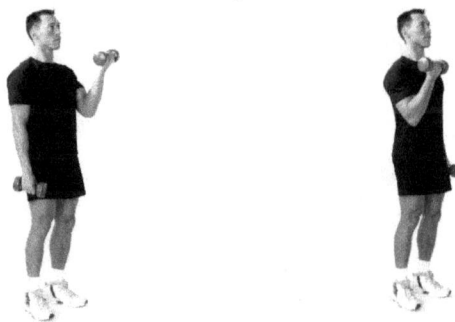

REVERSE BICEPS CURL
(BICEPS CURL
REVERSE GRIP)

Primary muscles:
Brachioradialis, brachialis,
biceps brachii

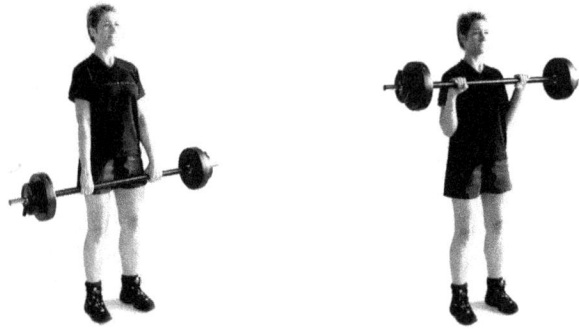

BICEPS DUMBBELL CURL

Primary muscles:
Biceps brachii, brachialis,
brachioradialis

BICEPS ALTERNATING
DUMBBELL CURL

Primary muscles:
Biceps brachii, brachialis,
brachioradialis

Standing. Contract the core muscles to stabilize the body. Grip barbell, underhand grip, slightly wider than shoulder-width. Bend the arms as much as possible without the elbow moving forward. Lower with control, arms straight, but not hyperextended.	Biceps barbell curl is the most direct biceps exercise, when performed with an underhand grip. Used for building muscle mass. Use full range of motion; all the way up working against gravity, and all the way down; elbows extend, but no hyperextension.	Different arm/body/leg position. Grip: Narrow (long head focus), medium, wide (short head focus). Note: Watch wrist and elbow when using a special grip. Different bars, such as an EZ-bar.
Standing. Contract the core muscles to stabilize the body. Grip barbell, overhand grip, hands slightly wider than shoulder-width apart. Bend the arms. Lower with control.	Focus on brachioradialis and brachialis. Strengthens the forearm muscles.	Different arm/body/leg position. Grip: Narrow (long head focus), medium, wide (short head focus). Note: Watch wrist and elbow when using a special grip. Different bars, such as an EZ-bar.
Standing. Contract the core muscles to stabilize the body. The arms at sides, a dumbbell in each hand. Palms face the body. Bend the arms at the same time and rotate, so the palms end up facing the chest. Elbows remain in place. Lower with control.	Avoid swinging the arms, control the movement. Contract the core muscles to stabilize the body.	Different arm/body/leg position. Standing, kneeling, sitting. Under, over- or neutral grip. If overhand grip, pronation, focus shifts from biceps to brachialis and brachioradialis.
Standing. Contract the core muscles to stabilize the body. The arms at sides, a dumbbell in each hand. Palms face the body. Bend and rotate one arm, so the palm faces the chest in top position. Alternate, repeat with the opposite arm, while lowering first arm with control.	You can alternate or work one arm at a time. One arm at a time works well for isolations, but keep contracting the 'resting' arm. Tip: Start the movement from top position, with both arms bent, then the top 'resting' arm is still contracted.	Different arm/body/leg position. Standing, sitting, kneeling. Under, over- or neutral grip.

BICEPS ALTERNATING DUMBBELL CURL Primary muscles: Biceps brachii, brachialis, brachioradialis	
BICEPS CURL IN BALANCE POSITION Primary muscles: Biceps brachii, brachialis, brachioradialis	
ZOTTMAN CURL Primary muscles: Biceps brachii, brachialis, brachioradialis	
BICEPS TUBE CURL ROTATED Primary muscles: Biceps brachii, brachialis, brachioradialis	

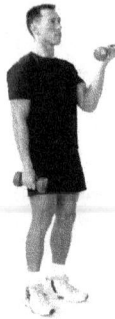

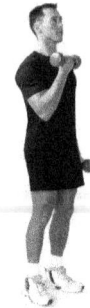

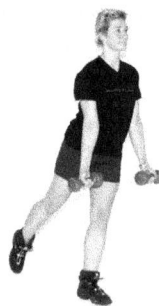

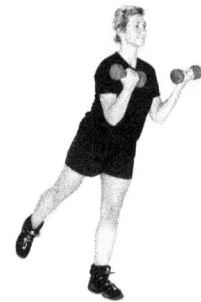

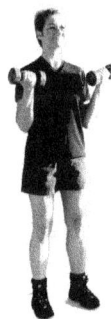

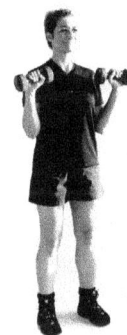

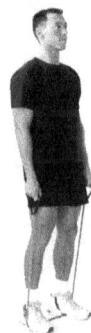

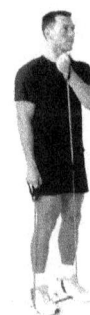

Standing. Contract the core muscles to stabilize the body. The arms at sides. A dumbbell in each hand. The palms face the body. The arms bend alternatingly and rotate, so the palms face the chest in top position. Elbows remain in place.	You can alternate or work one arm at a time. One arm at a time works well for isolations, but keep contracting the 'resting' arm. Tip: Start the movement from top position, with both arms bent, then the top 'resting' arm is still contracted.	Different arm/body/leg position. Standing, sitting, kneeling. Under, over- or neutral grip.
Standing on one leg. Contract the core muscles to stabilize the body. The arms at sides. A dumbbell in each hand, with an underhand grip. Bend the arms. Elbows remain in place. Lower.	Biceps curl with balance work. The torso can be erect or forward at different angles. Use full range of motion; bend arms all the way up, against gravity, and extend all the way down, elbows extend, but no hyperextension.	Different arm/body/leg position. Under, over- or neutral grip. If using an overhand grip, pronation, focus shifts from biceps to brachialis and brachioradialis.
Standing. Contract the core muscles to stabilize the body. The dumbbells in the hands, held with an underhand grip. 1. The arms bend to top position. 2. Turn the hands in the top, overhand grip. 3. Lower the arms with control. 4. Turn the hands back, underhand grip.	Avoid swinging the arms, keep the movement under control. Contract the core muscles to stabilize the body. Note: Only phase 1 and 2 are shown on the photo.	Different arm/body/leg position.
Standing. Contract the core muscles to stabilize the body. The arms at sides. A dumbbell in each hand. Bend one arm at a time. The arm rotates, so it bends close in front of the body, not forward in the sagittal plane. Palm moves toward the chin. Lower with control.	Resist the downward part, the eccentric phase, of the exercise.	Different arm/body/leg position.

EXERCISE	TECHNIQUE

**BICEPS CURL
PRONE INCLINE**

Primary muscles:
Biceps brachii, brachialis,
brachioradialis

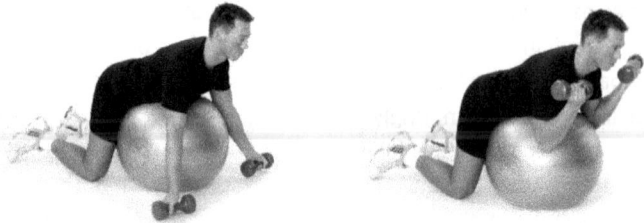

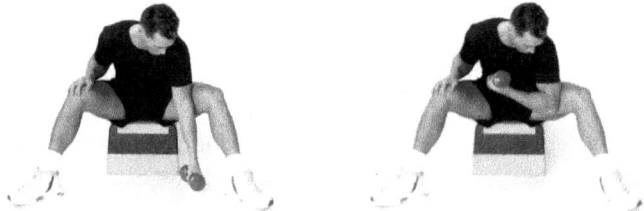

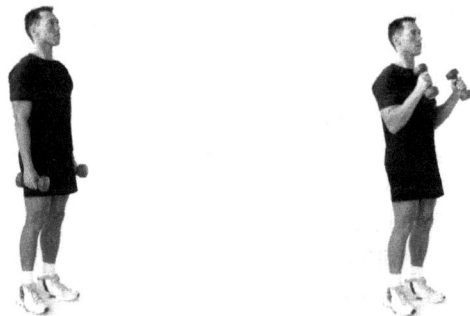

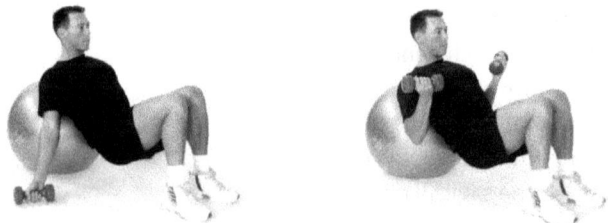

CONCENTRATION CURL

Primary muscles:
Biceps brachii, brachialis,
brachioradialis

HAMMER CURL

Primary muscles:
Biceps brachii, brachialis,
brachioradialis

INCLINE CURL

Primary muscles:
Biceps brachii, brachialis,
brachioradialis

Kneeling behind a ball. Ab/chest supported on ball. Grip dumbbell(s) with an underhand grip. If possible, keep upper arms off the ball (requires a big ball and a good balance). One or both arms bend. Lower with control.	Limited range of motion. The arms must hang free, vertical, to obtain the right effect in this exercise. Better variations: Standing, bent over with the head supported, or lying prone on an incline bench.	Different body/leg position. Unilateral, bilateral. With dumbbell(s) or barbell. A special bench is preferable to a ball, which makes full range of motion difficult to achieve.
Sitting. Legs wide. One upper arm supporting on the inside of one thigh. Dumbbell in hand. Palm face up towards the body, supinated. Bend arm, avoid swinging or assisting with the leg. Lower with control.	Try to increase the range of motion, extend the elbow completely, but without hyperextending the elbow.	**STANDING CONCENTRATION CURL** One arm bent at 90 degrees, across the waist, hand at the opposide side of the waist. The opposite arm, working arm rests on the hand. Bend the arm. Lower with control.
Standing. Contract the core muscles to stabilize the body. The arms at sides. A dumbbell in each hand. Palms face each other throughout the exercise. Elbows remains in place. Lower with control.	One arm may complete the exercise, or the other arm starts bending, when the first is in top position; alternating hammer curl. Avoid swinging the arms.	Different arm/body/leg position. Standing, sitting, kneeling.
Sitting, incline approx. 30 degrees, on ball or incline bench. Arms hang down, vertical position. They must hang freely, so the biceps brachii is fully stretched. Hands hold the dumbbells with an underhand grip. Bend the arms. Elbows remain in place. Lower.	The arms should be in vertical position with elbows extended. Use full range of motion in the elbow joint. Keep contracting during the eccentric phase. For isolation keep elbows in place. For shoulder work, move the arms forward in top position.	Different arm/body/leg position. One or both arms. On ball or bench.

PULL UP

Primary muscles:
Biceps brachii, brachialis,
latissimus dorsi

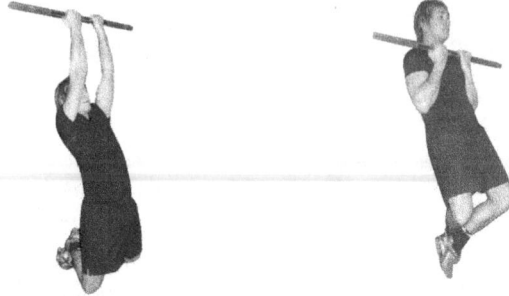

**TRICEPS (PUSH-UP)
STANDING (WALL/PARTNER)**

Primary muscles:
Triceps brachii, anterior
deltoid, pectoralis major

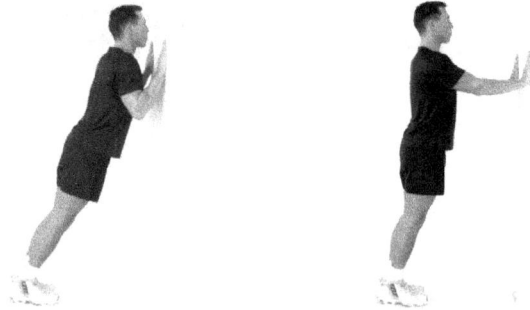

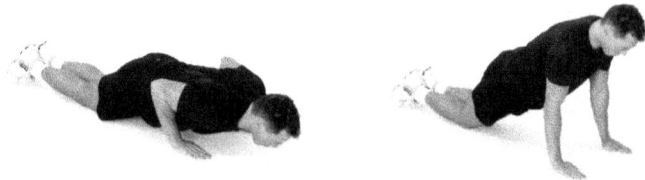

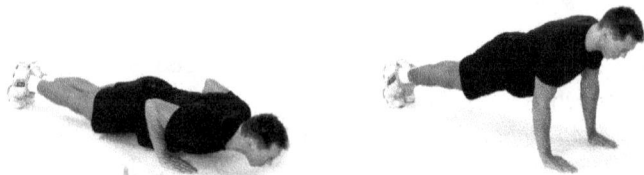

**TRICEPS PUSH-UP,
KNEELING**

Primary muscles:
Triceps brachii, anterior
deltoid, pectoralis major

**TRICEPS PUSH-UP,
PLANK POSITION (ON TOES)**

Primary muscles:
Triceps brachii, anterior
deltoid, pectoralis major

Hanging. Shoulder-width grip on bar or wall bar. Underhand grip. Pull the body up, until the chin is level with the bar or above. Lower with control, avoid going to far down and hyperextending the elbows.	For advanced exercisers. If you lack the strength to do a single pull up, start hanging with one leg supporting (pushing off) from a bench – or have a partner help lifting you.	Different arm position and grip. With or without support/help.
Standing. The hands support on wall, shoulder-width or narrower. Bend the arms, so the body is lowered towards the wall. Extend the arms, so the body Is pushed back to starting position. Move all of the body as a unit, not just the torso.	For beginners. Contract the core muscles to stabilize the body. Keep elbows straight backwards, upper arms close to the body, in the sagittal plane.	**INCLINE PUSH-UP** The hands on bench, ball, teeterboard ot the like. **STANDING PARTNER PUSH-UP** Face each other, the arms shoulder-width or wider – the palms against each other. Bend and extend the arms at the same time.
Plank position (short lever). Lower legs are on the floor or are lifted. The hands are on the floor, shoulder-width apart. Bend the arms, so the body is lowered towards the floor. Extend the arms, so the body is pushed back up.	Contract the core muscles to stabilize the body. Elbows point straight back, upper arms are kept close to the rib cage, in the sagittal plane. Stop when upper arms are parallel to the floor.	Different hand position. Different body position (more or less pike).
Plank position. On the hands and toes. The hands and arms are shoulder-width apart. Bend the arms, so all of the body, as one unit, is lowered towards the floor. Extend the arms, so the body is pushed back up.	Contract the core muscles to stabilize the body. Elbows point straight back, upper arms are kept close to the rib cage, in the sagittal plane. Stop when upper arms are parallel to the floor.	Different hand position. Different leg position (eg. One leg or legs narrow or wide). **COMBINATION EXERCISES** Change leg- or body position during the exercise.

DECLINE TRICEPS PUSH-UP

Primary muscles:
Triceps brachii, anterior
deltoid, pectoralis major

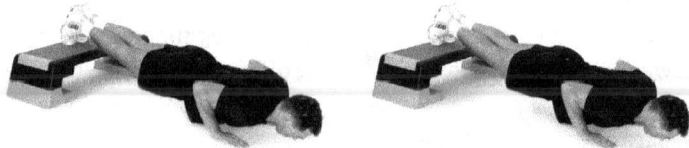

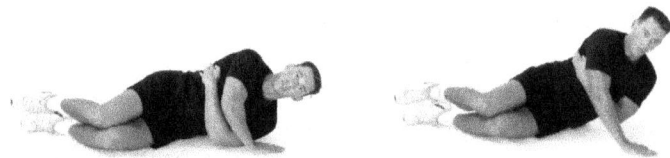

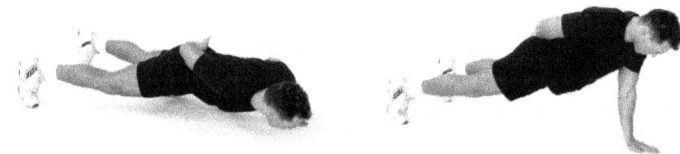

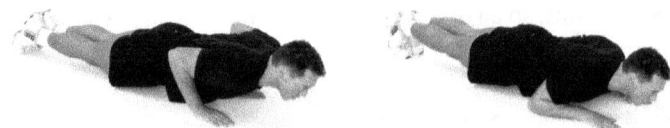

**TRICEPS ONE-ARM
PUSH-UP, SPECIAL
SIDELYING**

Primary muscles:
Triceps brachii, anterior
deltoid, pectoralis major

**TRICEPS ONE-ARM
PUSH-UP**

Primary muscles:
Triceps brachii, anterior
deltoid, pectoralis major

HINGE PUSH-UP

Primary muscles:
Triceps brachii, anterior
deltoid, pectoralis major

Plank position. On hands and toes. Feet on a bench (bench height may vary). Hands shoulder-width apart or narrower. Bend the arms, so all of the body, as one unit, is lowered towards the floor. Extend the arms to push the body back up.	For advanced exercisers. Contract the core muscles to stabilize the body. Elbows point straight back, upper arms are kept close to the rib cage, in the sagittal plane.	Different arm position. Different leg position.
Sidelying. Legs slightly bent. Top hand, working arm, is on the floor just below the shoulder. Other arm around the waist. Extend the working arm to push the body off the floor. Lower the body, stop just before the body rests on the floor.	Make the movement as large as possible, as range of motion is already limited. Extend the elbow, but no hyperextension. Bend/lower as far down as possible without resting on the floor.	**TRICEPS ONE-ARM SPECIAL PUSH-UP WITH TORSO ROTATION** Sidelying. Top hand on the floor. Free arm is forward just above the floor under the top arm. When pushing off, the body rotates backwards and free arm points to the back. Return to the starting point.
Plank position. On one hand and toes. The hand is on the floor just below the shoulder. Free arm position is optional. Bend the arm, so the body is lowered towards the floor. Extend the arm, so the body is pushed back up.	For advanced exercisers. Contract the core muscles to stabilize the body. Keep the shoulders and pelvis level. To learn the correct technique, start in an upright position and gradually lower your point of support. Or with a partner holding a towel around the waist or holding the shoulders.	Different arm position. Different leg position (eg. on one leg, or legs narrow or wide position).
Plank position. On the hands and toes. Push-up with four phases: 1) Bend, go down, 2) push the body backwards, down onto your forearms, 3) lift slightly and move forward, 4) extend arms, push back up.	For advanced exercisers. All four phases should be performed. Contract the core muscles to stabilize the body. Start on the top, dorsal side, of your foot, so you are able to move the body backwards.	On one or both arms. Different leg position.

**TRICEPS PUSH-UP
HANDS STAGGERED**

Primary muscles:
Triceps brachii, anterior
deltoid, pectoralis major

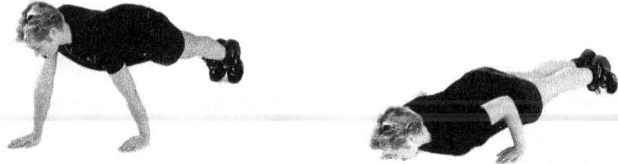

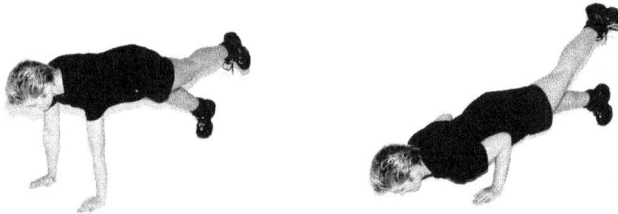

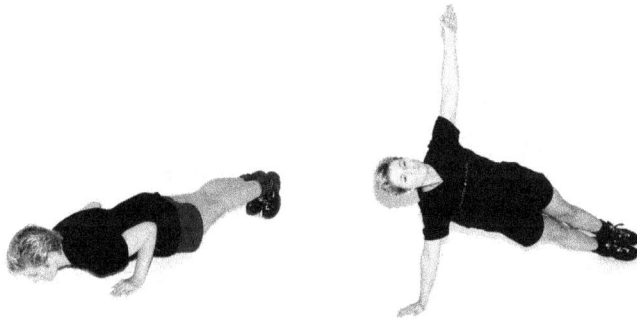

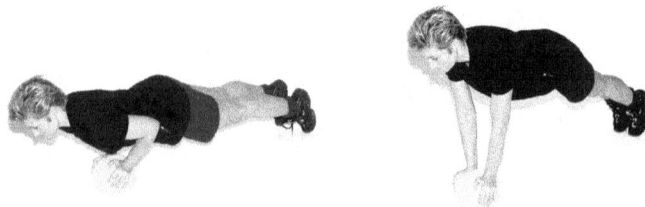

**TRICEPS PUSH-UP
ON ONE LEG**

Primary muscles:
Triceps brachii, anterior
deltoid, pectoralis major

**TRICEPS
T-PUSH-UP**

Primary muscles:
Triceps brachii, anterior
deltoid, pectoralis major

**TRICEPS
PUSH-UP HANDS NARROW,
ON BALL**

Primary muscles:
Triceps brachii, anterior
deltoid, pectoralis major

Plank position. On the hands and toes. Hands are staggered forward/backward. Bend the arms, so the body is lowered towards the floor. Extend the arms, so the body is pushed up.	Contract the core muscles to stabilize the body. Triceps push-up variation for continued stimulation. Remember to change arms, so you work both arms in the same way.	Different leg position.
Plank position. On the hands and one foot. Other leg is lifted off the floor. Bend the arms, lower the body. Extend the arms, so the body is pushed back up.	For intermediate exercisers. Contract the core muscles to stabilize the body. Neck in neutral position. Triceps push-up with balance work.	On one or both arms. Different leg position.
Plank position. On the hands and toes. Hands shoulder-width apart. Bend the arms, so the body is lowered towards the floor. Extend the arms and turn the body to one side into a one-arm side support. Repeat to the opposite side.	For intermediate exercises. Contract the core muscles to stabilize the body. Elbows point straight to the back, upper arms are kept close to the rib cage. Triceps push-up with balance and core work.	Different leg position (eg. top leg lifts).
Plank position. On the hands and toes. Hands together on a medicine ball (or other small ball). Bend the arms, so the body is lowered towards the floor. Extend the arms, so the body is pushed back up.	For advanced exercisers. Contract the core muscles to stabilize the body. Elbows point straight to the back, upper arms are kept close to the rib cage, Triceps push-up with balance work.	Different arm position. Different leg position.

EXERCISE	TECHNIQUE

LATERAL PUSH-UP

Primary muscles:
Triceps brachii, anterior
deltoid, pectoralis major

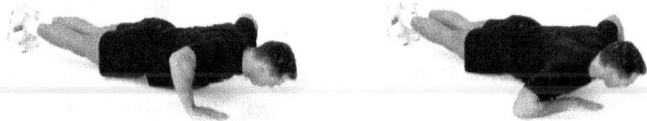

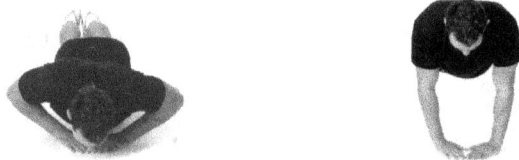

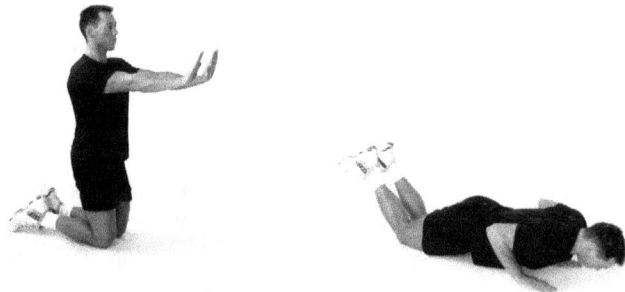

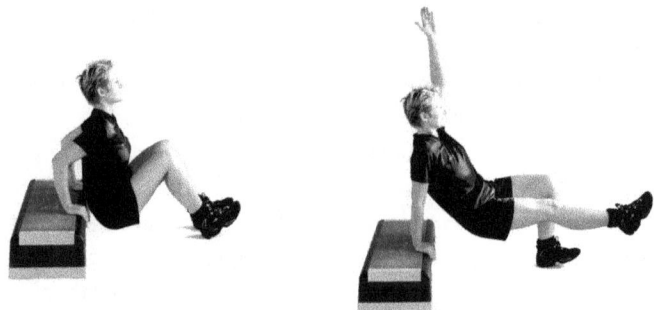

TRICEPS PUSH-UP, NARROW

Primary muscles:
Triceps brachii, anterior
deltoid, pectoralis major

**PLYOMETRIC PUSH-UP
FREE FALL ON KNEES**

Primary muscles:
Triceps brachii, anterior
deltoid pectoralis major

TRICEPS DIP ON BENCH

Primary muscles:
Triceps brachii, anterior
deltoid, pectoralis major

TECHNIQUE	FOCUS	VARIATION
Plank position. On the hands and toes. The arms wide apart. Hands point slightly inwards. Push-up with four phases: 1) Bend, 2) push the body out to one side and down on the forearm, 3) push back to center, 4) extend, push back up to starting position.	For advanced exercisers. Perform all four phases with control and precision. Contract the core muscles to stabilize the body.	On one or both arms. Different leg position.
Plank position. On the hands and lower legs (or toes). Thumbs and indexfingers of both hands touch each other, elbows slightly outwards. Bend the arms, so the body is lowered towards the floor. Extend the arms, so the body is pushed back up.	For advanced exercisers. Contract the core muscles to stabilize the body. Keep elbows pointing in the same direction as the hands.	Different arm position. Different leg position.
Kneeling (or standing). Torso upright, hips straight. Arms forward, shoulder level, in front of the chest. Free-fall down into push-up. Break the fall with the arms. Push the body back up to the starting position. Either with the arms alone or with a little help from the body (hips).	For advanced exercisers. Watch the wrists. Build strength gradually with a small range of motion and few repetitions and land on a mat. Advanced exercisers may (with years of basic training) free-fall from a standing position. Contract the core muscles to stabilize the body.	**PUSH-UP WITH CLAP** Forcefully push off floor, clap hands, while in the air. Land. **DEPTH PUSH-UP** Feet on floor or bench, the arms wide on a bench each. Free-fall down to the floor between benches. Power push back up.
Sitting on a bench. Hands on the bench with fingers pointing forward off the edge, so the wrists must not bend as much. Body is off the bench, buttocks close to the bench. Feet on the floor. Bend the arms and lower the body. Extend the arms, then lift one arm and opposite leg. Repeat with opposite side.	For balance work. Keep the shoulders down and the neck 'long'. The movement should be in the elbows, and shoulders, and have some range of motion. Note: The exercise is hard on the shoulder ligaments.	Progression. 1. Triceps dip. Both hands on bench, both feet on the floor. 2. From dip extend arms, lift one arm, one hand supports. 3. From dip to one arm, lift leg (same side as supporting arm). Vary foot distance from bench. Different leg position (one leg, both legs, crossovers).

EXERCISE	TECHNIQUE

**TRICEPS DIP ON BENCH
WITH BARBELL**

Primary muscles:
Triceps brachii, anterior
deltoid, pectoralis major

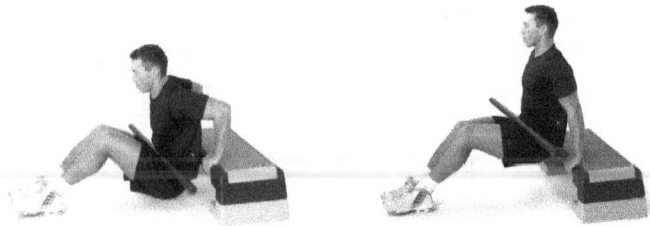

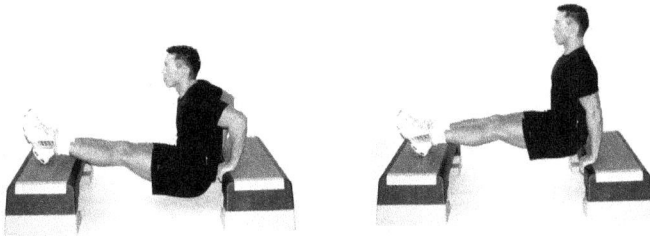

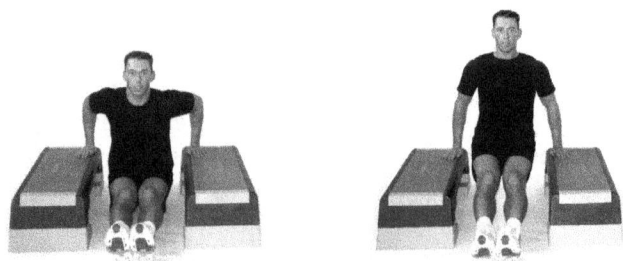

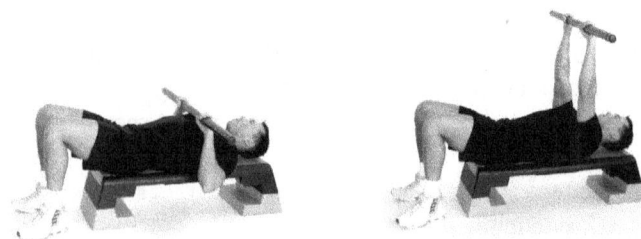

**TRICEPS DIP ON
TWO BENCHES**

Primary muscles:
Triceps brachii, anterior
deltoid, pectoralis major

**TRICEPS DIP BETWEEN
TWO BENCHES**

Primary muscles:
Triceps brachii, anterior
deltoid, pectoralis major

**BENCH PRESS,
NARROW GRIP**

Primary muscles:
Triceps brachii, anterior
deltoid, pectoralis major

Sitting on bench. Fingers off the edge, which is easier on the wrists. Legs slightly bent. Barbell on thighs. Buttocks are close to the bench and feet are on the floor. Shoulders down. Bend the arms and lower the body. Extend the arms again, but avoid hyper-extending the elbows.	Keep the shoulders down, so the neck is 'long'. The movement should be in the elbows, and the shoulders, – with some range of motion. Note: The exercise is hard on the shoulders and the wrists. Not for recommended if you have shoulder problems.	Legs bent or straight, different points of support. Different leg position (one leg, both legs, crossed legs, combinations). With barbell or medicine ball.
Sitting on a bench. Hands on one bench, fingers pointing forward. Fingers off the edge; easier on the wrists. Body between benches, buttocks close to the bench. Feet are on the other bench. Shoulders down. Bend the arms and lower the body. Extend arms, return to starting position.	Keep the shoulders down, so the neck is 'long' and away from the shoulders. The movement should be in the elbows and shoulders – not the buttom going up and down – have some range of motion. Note: The exercise is hard on the shoulders and the wrists.	Legs bent or straight, different points of support. Different leg position (eg. one leg, both legs, crossed legs, combinations). With or without barbell.
Sitting between two benches. The hands on a bench each with the fingers forward. The body is lifted, the heels are on the floor. The shoulders are down. The arms bend and the body is lowered. Extend the arms, return to starting position.	Keep the shoulders down, so the neck is 'long' and away from the shoulders. The movement should be in the elbows and shoulders – not the buttom going up and down – have some range of motion. Note: The exercise is hard on the shoulders and the wrists.	Legs bent or straight, different points of support. Different leg position (eg. one leg, both legs, crossed legs, combinations).
Supine on bench. Hands hold the barbell. Hands shoulder-width apart. Press the barbell straight up above the chest. As a benchpres, but narrow grip for a triceps focus. The arms move close to the torso, rib cage, in the sagittal plane. Wrists are in neutral.	Barbell just above the forearm. Keep the wrists neutral, do not bend (extend) backwards, so the barbell pull on the wrists.	Different leg position.

EXERCISE	TECHNIQUE

FRENCH PRESS

Primary muscles:
Triceps brachii

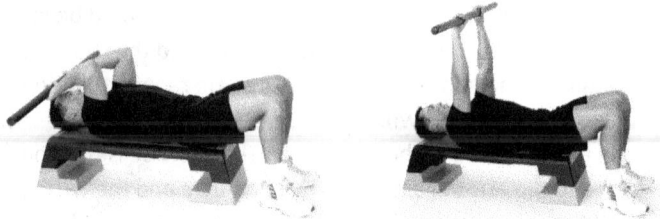

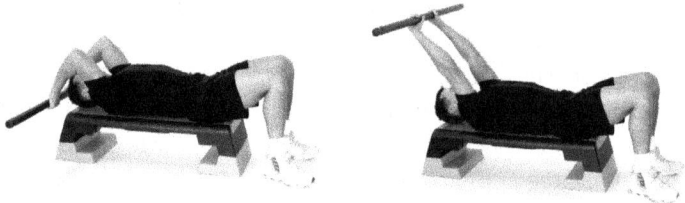

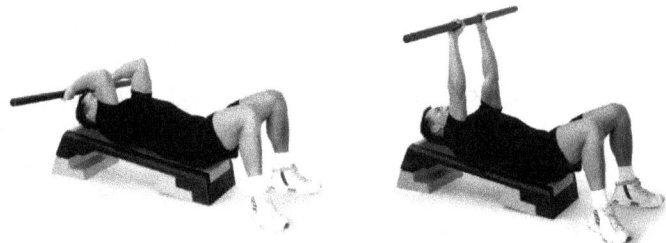

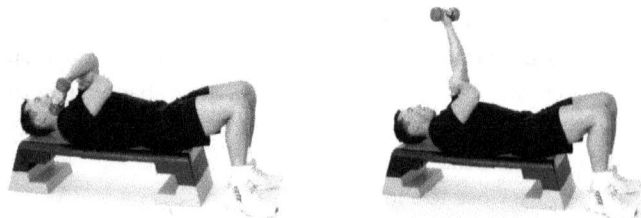

FRENCH PRESS, 45 DEGREES

Primary muscles:
Triceps brachii

FRENCH PRESS, INCLINE

Primary muscles:
Triceps brachii

**LYING CROSS FACE
TRICEPS EXTENSION**

Primary muscles:
Triceps brachii

Supine. Hands hold the barbell, shoulder-width apart. Arms vertical, perpendicular to body. The wrists are neutral. Bend the arms, so the barbell is lowered to a point just behind the forehead. Extend the arms, using the triceps, do not pull with the shoulders.	Control the movement – use a spotter. No shoulder movement. The movement is in the elbows. Hold dumbbell/barbell over the forearm. Keep wrists in neutral position. Do not let the barbell pull on the wrists.	Different leg position. Over-, under-, neutral grip. On floor, bench or ball. Flat, incline or decline bench. With dumbbells, barbell or medicine ball.
Supine. The hands hold the barbell, shoulder-width apart. Arms are straight and back, 45 degrees. Wrists are straight. Bend the arms, so the barbell is lowered to a point behind the head, forearm vertical. Extend the arms, using the triceps; do not pull with the shoulders.	Control the movement – use a spotter. No shoulder movement. The movement is in the elbows. Hold dumbbell/barbell over the forearm. Keep wrists in neutral position. Do not let the barbell pull on the wrists.	Different leg position. Over-, under-, neutral grip. On floor, bench or ball. Flat, incline or decline bench. With dumbbells, barbell or medicine ball.
Supine on incline bench, with dumbbells or a barbell. Arms straight, vertical position. Bend the arms, so the barbell is lowered to the forehead, or a little behind the forehead. Extend the arms, using the triceps; do not pull with the shoulders.	Control the movement – use a spotter. No shoulder movement. The movement is in the elbows. Hold dumbbell/barbell over the forearm. Keep wrists in neutral position. Do not let the barbell pull on the wrists.	Different leg position. Over-, under-, neutral grip. With dumbbells, barbell or medicine ball.
Supine on bench. One arm vertical with a dumbbell in the hand. Opposite hand stabilizes the working arm. Bend the working arm, so the dumbbell is lowered to the opposite shoulder. Extend the arm, using the triceps, do not pull with the shoulder.	Control the movement – use a spotter. No shoulder movement. The movement is in the elbow. Keep wrist in neutral position. Do not let the dumbbell pull on the wrist.	Different leg position. On floor, bench or ball.

EXERCISE	TECHNIQUE

TRICEPS EXTENSION HIGH, FACE-AWAY

Primary muscles:
Triceps brachii,
anterior deltoid

TRICEPS OVERHEAD EXTENSION

Primary muscles:
Triceps brachii

TRICEPS KICK BACK

Primary muscles:
Triceps brachii,
posterior deltoid

TRICEPS KICK BACK, ONE-ARM, KNEELING

Primary muscles:
Triceps brachii,
posterior deltoid

Standing. Legs staggered. Band anchored behind the body (high position). Upper arms are at or above horizontal, the hands hold the band. Extend the arms, forearms in line with upper arms, to pull the tube forward. Return with control.	Contract the core muscles to stabilize the body. Upper arms steady, movement is in the elbows.	Different body/leg position. Standing, sitting, kneeling. Over-, under-, neutral grip.
Standing. Torso erect. Upper arm(s) vertical. The hands together, holding a dumbbell, barbell or tube. Bend the arms, lower with control. Extend the arms back up.	Avoid pausing in the end ranges of the movement. Avoid 'locking' the elbows. Contract the core muscles to stabilize the body. Upper arms steady, movement is in the elbows.	Different body/leg position. Standing, sitting, kneeling. Unilateral, bilateral. Over-, under-, neutral grip. With a dumbbell or barbell, tube or band. With rubberband anchored on same side shoulder.
Standing. Feet staggered, the torso slightly forward. Upper arm(s) behind the body (shoulder extension). The hand(s) hold the weight (tube/band). Extend arm(s) with control – extend elbow(s) completely. Return with control	Contract the core muscles to stabilize the body. Upper arm steady, movement is in the elbows. Do not let the forearm go past vertical, as you stop working against gravity.	Different body/leg position. Standing, sitting, kneeling. Unilateral, bilateral. Over-, under-, neutral grip. With a dumbbell or barbell, tube or band. With rubberband anchored on same side hip.
Kneeling. One leg kneeling on a bench. Other leg off bench with foot on the floor. Hand supports on the bench to stabilize the body. Working arm above horizontal (shoulder extension). Extend elbow completely. Bend elbow approx. 90 degr. to lower forearm close to vertical.	Working arm above horizontal. Do not let the forearm go past vertical, as you stop working against gravity. Keep shoulders and hips level, do not rotate the body.	Different body/leg position. Unilateral, bilateral. Over-, under-, neutral grip. With dumbbell or barbell.

EXERCISE	TECHNIQUE

**TRICEPS PUSHDOWN
(PRESSDOWN)
WITH BAND/TUBE**

Primary muscles:
Triceps brachii

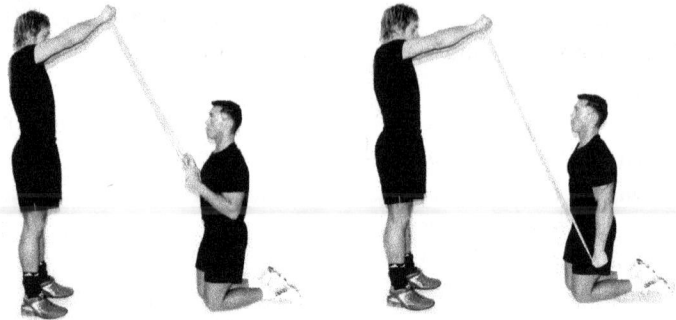

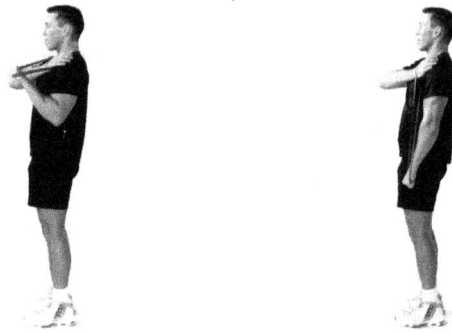

**TRICEPS PUSHDOWN
WITH RUBBERBAND**

Primary muscles:
Triceps brachii

**FOREARM CURL,
STANDING
(BEHIND THE BACK WRIST
CURL)**

Primary muscles:
Forearm flexors

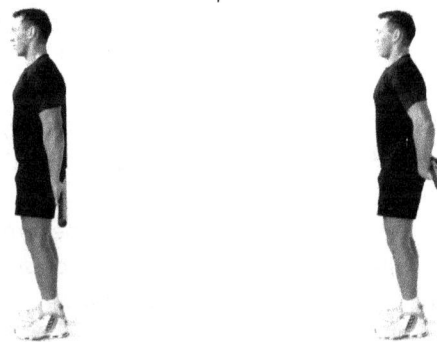

**FOREARM CURL,
OVERHAND GRIP
(REVERSE WRIST CURL)**

Primary muscles:
Forearm extensors

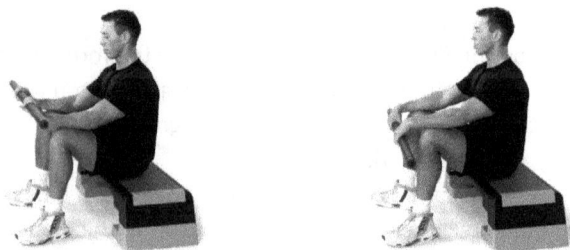

Standing (or kneeling with partner). A partner (or wall bar) anchors the band at a high position. Contract the core muscles to stabilize the body. Upper arms at sides. Extend the arms with control, full range of motion in the elbow. Return with control. Upper arms do not move.	Full range of motion: Extend the arms completely and let the elbows bend to full flexion controlling the movement with the triceps. Do not stop the forearms in horizontal position (a common mistake) as range of motion is reduced and the effect is lessened.	Different body/leg position. Standing or kneeling. Unilateral, bilateral. Over-, under-, neutral grip. With tube or band. **REVERSE PUSHDOWN** Triceps pushdown with an underhand grip.
Standing. Contract the core muscles to stabilize the body. One hand on the shoulder, holding the rubberband. Opposite hand grips the band. Extend working arm, push down against the rubberband. Return with control.	Contract the core to stabilize. Upper arm stays in the same position, the movement is in the elbow. Mind the wrist, keep it in neutral position.	Different body/leg position. Standing, sitting, kneeling. Over-, under-, neutral grip. With rubberband, tube or band.
Standing. Barbell behind the body. Hands hold the barbell with an underhand grip, palms face away from the body. Open the fingers and let the barbell slide down a little. Close the fingers around the bar again and curl the wrist upwards.	Note: Be careful not to drop the barbell.	Different body/leg position. **FOREARM CURL** Sitting. Forearms on legs. Underhand grip on barbell. Lower barbell by bending the wrist backwards (extend) and let the fingers open, so the barbell rolls down into the fingers. Bend fingers again, bend wrist and return.
Sitting on bench. Forearms on the legs. Overhand grip on the barbell. Lift the barbell by extending the wrists, bending the hands as far back as possible. Lower with control.	Note: Be careful not to drop the barbell.	Sitting on bench or ball.

**WRIST EXTENSION
WITH THERA-BAND®
SOFTWEIGHT BALL**

Primary muscles:
Forearm extensor muscles

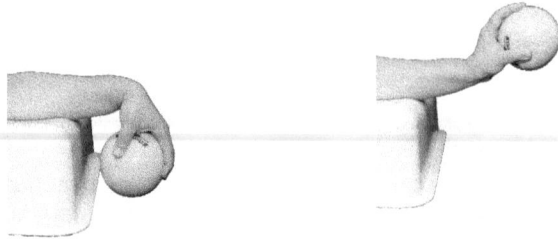

**WRIST FLEXION
WITH THERA-BAND®
SOFTWEIGHT BALL**

Primary muscles:
Forearm flexor muscles

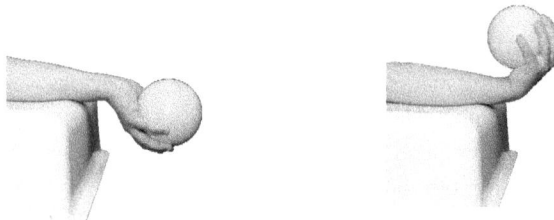

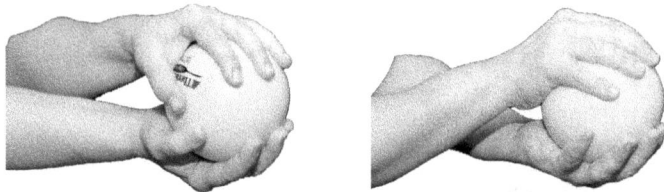

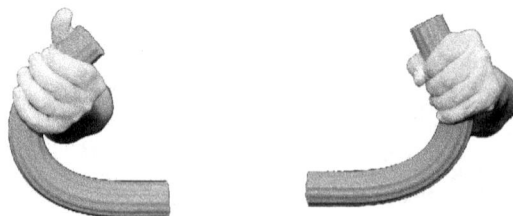

**FOREARM ROTATION
WITH THERA-BAND®
SOFTWEIGHT BALL**

Primary muscles:
Forearm muscles

**FOREARM ROTATION
WITH THERA-BAND®
FLEXBAR**

Primary muscles:
Forearm muscles

Forearm on a table edge, hand with palm downwards. Thera-Band Softweight ball in the hand. Lift and lower the hand with the Thera-Band Softweight ball as resistance. 	Exercising with a ball is a super workout for the forearm and finger muscles. Balls comes in different sizes (and weights).	Different arm- and hand positions.
Forearm on a table edge, hand with palm upwards. Thera-Band Softweight ball in the hand. Lift and lower the hand with the Thera-Band Softweight ball as resistance. 	Exercising with a ball is a super workout for the forearm and finger muscles. Balls comes in different sizes (and weights).	Different arm- and hand positions.
Hold a Thera-Band Softweight ball with both hands. Right and left hand changes place, so they alternate from top to bottom position. 	Exercising with a ball is a super workout for the forearm and finger muscles. Balls comes in different sizes (and weights).	Different arm- and hand positions.
Hold one end of a Thera-Band FlexBar. Press the other end down into the table. At the same time turn the palm towards the table. Repeat, but this time turn the palm up. 	The FlexBar can be used for a range of different forearm exercises.	Different arm- and hand positions.

EXERCISE	TECHNIQUE

**HAND SQUEEZE
WITH THERA-BAND®
HAND TRAINER**

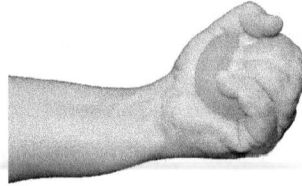

Primary muscles:
Finger flexors muscles

**HAND ROLL
WITH THERA-BAND®
HAND TRAINER**

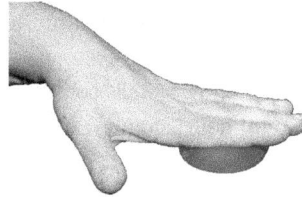

Primary muscles:
Finger extensor muscles

**HAND SQUEEZE ON
NCM THERA-PUTTY™**

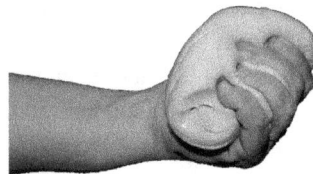

Primary muscles:
Finger flexor muscles

**FINGER EXTENSION WITH
NCM THERA-PUTTY™**

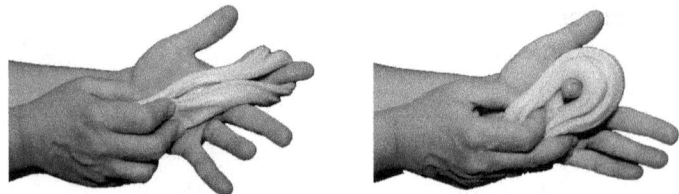

Primary muscles:
Finger extensor muscles

Hold a Thera-Band Hand Trainer in the hand. Palm faces upwards. Alternate between squeezing the Hand Trainer and relaxing the grip. Move the Hand Trainer during the exercise. 	Balls come with different levels of resistance.	Different finger movements. With all of the hand or just one finger at a time.
Roll Thera-Band Hand Trainer on a table or smooth surface. Roll back and forth, from side to side, while pressing down on the Hand Trainer at the same time. 	Balls come with different levels of resistance.	Different finger movements. With all of the hand or just one finger at a time.
Place NCM TheraPutty in the palm and press the fingers into the putty, until they touch the palm. Clench the hand completely. Relax the fingers again and roll the putty in the hand. Repeat. 	The putty can be used for several hand exercises, and provides a good finger workout, as it is quite demanding to mold the putty.	Different finger movements. With all of the hand or just one finger at a time.
Bend a finger, so the tip of the finger is close to the palm of the hand. Put a loop of NCM TheraPutty around the finger. Extend the finger against the resistance. Repeat with all the fingers. 	The putty can be used for several hand exercises, and provides a good finger workout, as it is quite demanding to mold the putty.	Different finger movements. With all of the hand or just one finger at a time.

7 | Hip and Leg Exercises

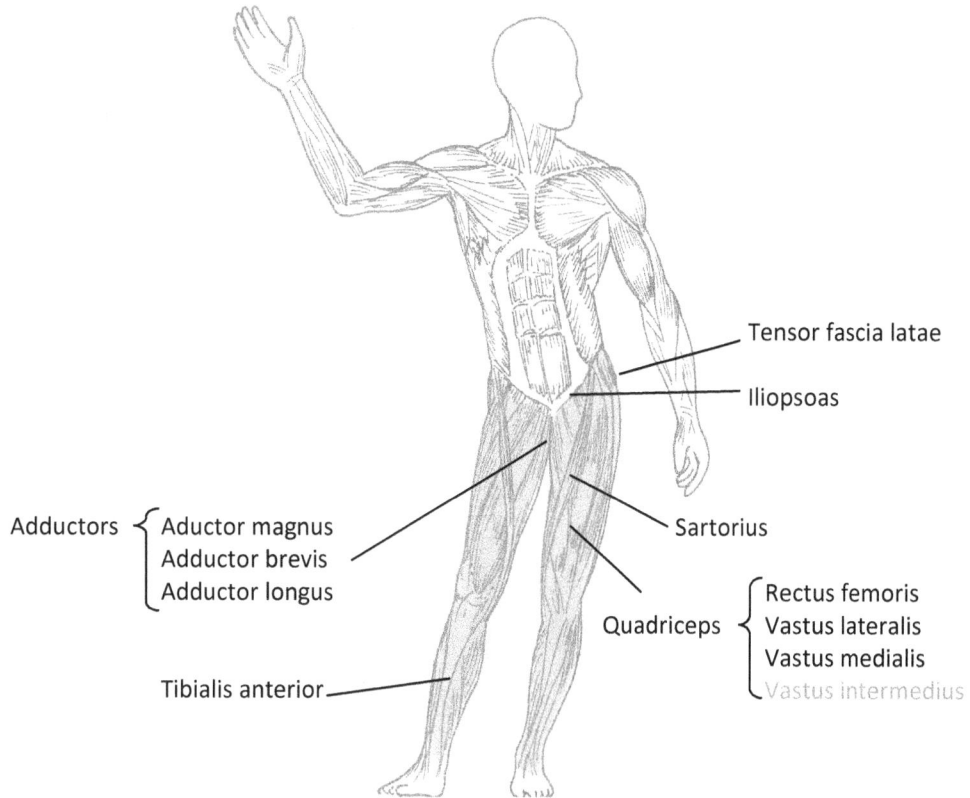

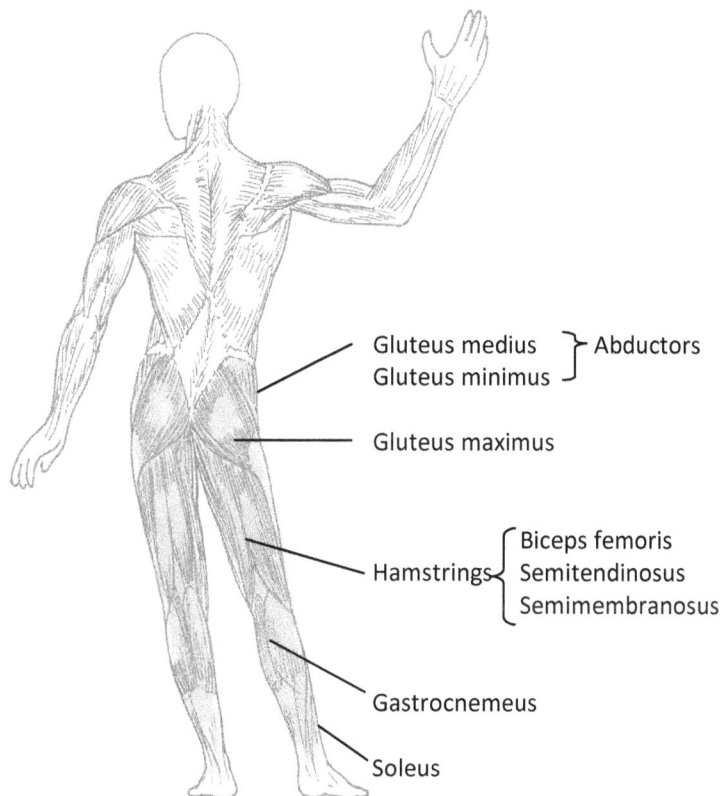

Tensor fascia latae

Iliopsoas

Adductors { Aductor magnus
Adductor brevis
Adductor longus

Sartorius

Quadriceps { Rectus femoris
Vastus lateralis
Vastus medialis
Vastus intermedius

Tibialis anterior

Gluteus medius ⎫ Abductors
Gluteus minimus ⎭

Gluteus maximus

Hamstrings { Biceps femoris
Semitendinosus
Semimembranosus

Gastrocnemeus

Soleus

THREE LEGGED LUNGE

Primary muscles:
Quadriceps,
gluteus maximus,
hamstrings

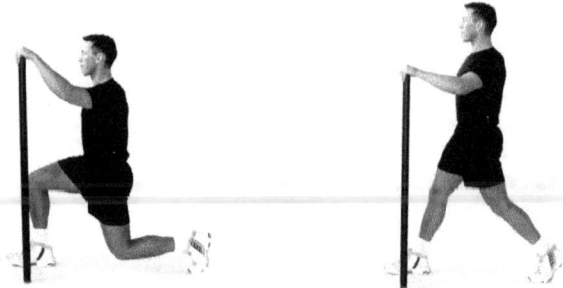

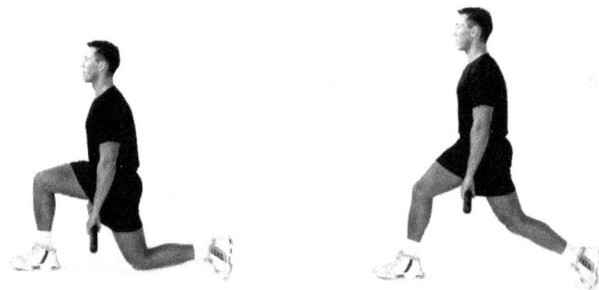

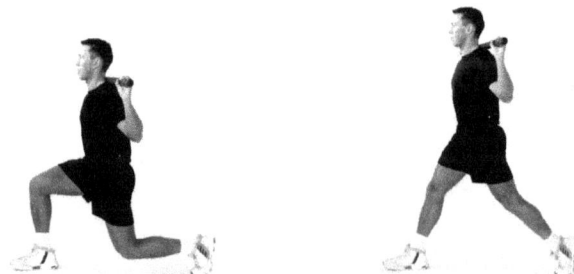

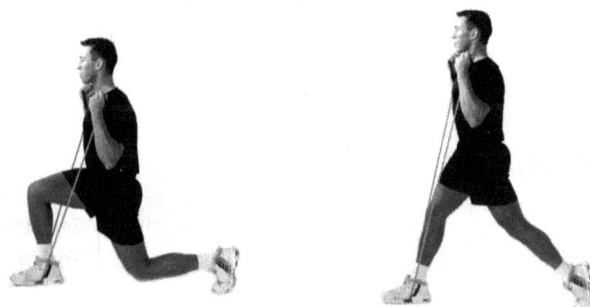

STATIONARY LUNGE, WIDE WITH BARBELL

Primary muscles:
Quadriceps,
gluteus maximus, hamstrings

SPLIT SQUAT (STATIONARY LUNGE)

Primary muscles:
Quadriceps,
gluteus maximus, hamstrings

LUNGE, STATIONARY, WIDE WITH TUBE/BAND

Primary muscles:
Quadriceps,
gluteus maximus, hamstrings

TECHNIQUE	NOTE	VARIATION
Standing. Feet staggered. Barbell on floor, in line with back foot and by the side of front foot, held with opposite arm. Bodyweight is between the legs. Stationary lunge: Bend legs with control to approx. 90 degrees flexion of both knees. Extend the knees, straigthen legs and return up.	Exercise for beginners and intermediate exercises. Check that both knees are in the right position and aligned with the feet. Focus on both the concentric and the eccentric phase of the exercise.	Shift the bodyweight. Eg. have most of the weight on the front foot to focus on the front leg muscles.
Standing. Feet staggered. Barbell between legs directly under the torso. Hold the barbel with the hands on each side of the body. Stationary lunge: Bend legs with control to approx. 90 degr. flexion in both knees. Extend the knees, straighten legs, and return up.	Special lunge, which will aid in remembering to keep torso upright. For beginners. Contract the core muscles to stabilize the body. Check that both knees are in the right position and aligned with the feet.	Different leg position and range of motion.
Standing. Feet staggered. With or without a barbell. Torso erect. Look forward. Stationary lunge: Bend legs with control to approx. 90 degrees flexion in both knees. Extend the knees, straighten legs, and return up.	Contract the core muscles to stabilize the body. Check that both knees are in the right position and aligned with the feet. Focus on both the concentric and the eccentric phase.	With or without resistance. With weight plate/medicine ball held close to the chest. With a barbell. With dumbbells.
Standing. Feet staggered. Tube or band under the front foot. Hold tube/band anchored at the shoulders with the hands. Stationary lunge: Bend legs with control to approx. 90 degree flexion in both knees. Extend the knees, straighten the legs, and return up.	Contract the core muscles to stabilize the body. Check that both knees are in the right position and aligned with the feet. Pay equal attention to the concentric and the eccentric phase of the exercise.	With tube or band. With front or back foot on a bench.

EXERCISE	TECHNIQUE

LUNGE

Primary muscles:
Gluteus maximus, hamstrings,
quadriceps

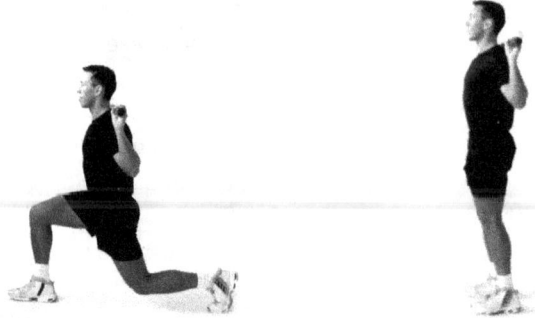

REAR LUNGE

Primary muscles:
Quadriceps,
gluteus maximus, hamstrings

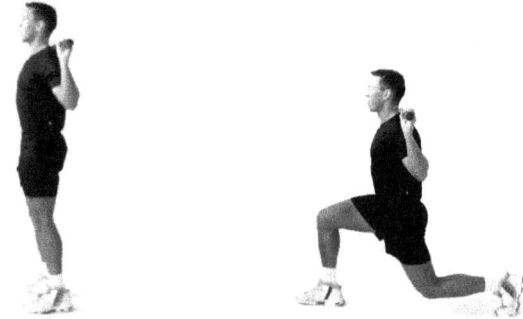

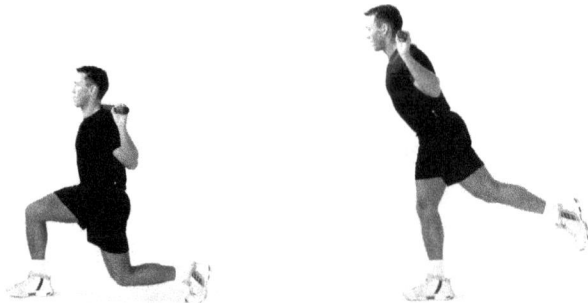

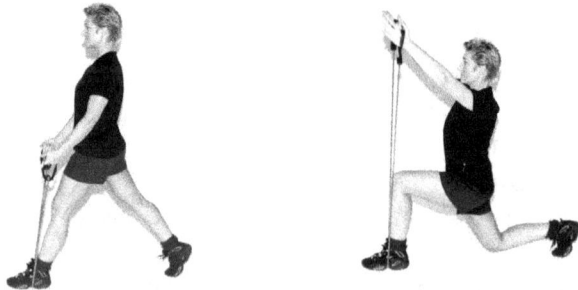

**REAR LUNGE
WITH HIP EXTENSION**

Primary muscles:
Quadriceps,
gluteus maximus, hamstrings

**STATIONARY LUNGE
WITH FRONT RAISE
WITH TUBE**

Primary muscles:
Quadriceps,
gluteus maximus, hamstrings

Standing. Feet hip-width apart. Take a large step forward; front foot land firmly on the floor. Front lower leg is vertical, back lower leg horizontal. Control the movement. Contract buttock and thigh and push/step back again. Repeat with the opposite leg.	Excellent functional exercise. Check that both knees are forward and aligned with feet. 90 degree angle in both knees. Optional: A longer step, more work, but is hard on hip. Gluteus focus: Push off with the heel of the the front leg. Requires some hamstring and adductor flexibility.	With or without resistance/ barbell. With rubberband/ resistance anchored behind the body and around the waist. **OVERHEAD LUNGE** Barbell in hands extended over the head **BOX LUNGE** Lunge up on a bench, 10-20 cm high. Step back. Different range of motion.
Standing. Feet hip-width apart Take a large step backward. Step with care. Front lower vertical, back lower leg around horizontal. Contract buttock and thigh and step forward, back to the start. Repeat with the opposite leg.	Check floor behind you. Even if a step backward is considered more difficult (than forward) a rear lunge may be a good alternative for beginners: Rear lunge reduces the risk of bending front knee too much. Requires some hamstring and adductor flexibility.	Different arm positions. Different arm exercises. With or without resistance/medicine ball. **LUNGE W/TORSOROTATION** When in lunge position, the torso rotates to the same side as the front leg. Return.
Standing. Feet hip-width apart. 1) Take a large step backward. Extend the front leg and 2) lift back leg back and up into hip extension. 3) Lower back down into lunge position, 4) step forward again. Repeat with the opposite leg.	Four phases. Check that both knees are in the right position and aligned with the feet. Contract the core muscles to stabilize the body. Requires some hamstring and adductor flexibility.	Different arm position. With or without barbell/ dumbbells/medicine ball.
Standing. Feet staggered, forward/backward, wide apart. 90 degree angle in both knees (on photo back knee over 90). Tube held under front foot. The handles in the hands. Bend down into lunge, at the same time lift the hands into front raise or high front raise. Extend knees and lower arms.	Check that both knees are in the right position and aligned with the feet. Pay equal attention to the concentric and the eccentric phase of the exercise. Tube provides resistance to the lunge and the front raise.	Different arm position. Different angle in knees.

EXERCISE	TECHNIQUE

LUNGE, NARROW

Primary muscles:
Quadriceps,
gluteus maximus, hamstrings
(focus quadriceps)

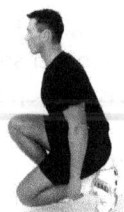

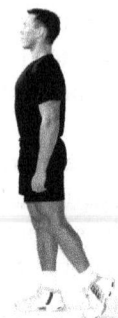

**LUNGE, NARROW
WITH HIP EXTENSION**

Primary muscles:
Gluteus maximus, hamstrings,
quadriceps

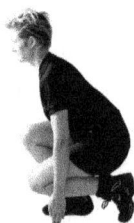

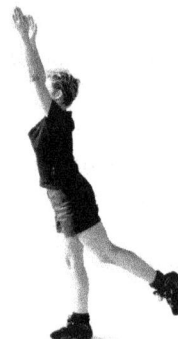

**LUNGE, NARROW
(UNI-SQUAT) UNSUPPORTED
WITH HIP EXTENSION**

Primary muscles:
Quadriceps,
gluteus maximus, hamstrings

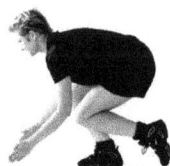

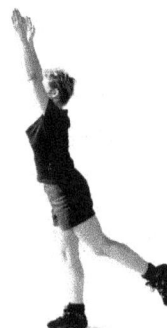

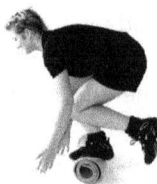

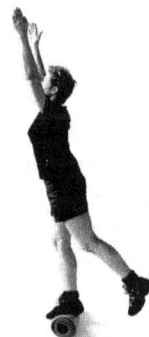

**LUNGE, NARROW
(UNI-SQUAT) ON UNSTABLE
SURFACE,
WITH HIP EXTENSION**

Primary muscles:
Quadriceps,
gluteus maximus, hamstrings

TECHNIQUE	NOTE	VARIATION
Standing. Feet staggered, hip-width apart, narrow stance. Bodyweight centered over front leg, back toe touch floor for balance. Bend down, deep flexion. Keep the torso is erect as possible. Extend legs, return back up.	Check that both knees are in the right position and aligned with the feet. Focus equally on the concentric and the eccentric phases of the exercise.	Different arm position. Stationary or with legs alternating (hop or step to change leg). With or without resistance/barbell.
Standing. Feet staggered, narrow stance. Bodyweight centered over front leg, back toe touch floor for balance. Bend down, deep flexion. Keep the torso erect. Extend legs, go up, lift back leg back into hip extension.	Check that both knees are in the right position and aligned with the feet. Focus equally on the concentric and the eccentric phase of the exercise.	Different arm position. Differentt range of motion.
Standing. Feet staggered, narrow stance. Bodyweight centered over front leg, back foot lifted just above the floor. Bend down, deep flexion. Keep the torso as erect as possible. Extend front leg, go up, and lift back leg back into hip extension.	For intermediate exercisers. Check that both knees are in the right position and aligned with the feet. Focus equally on the concentric and the eccentric phase of the exercise.	Different arm position. With or without movement of the free leg.
Standing. Feet staggered, narrow stance. Front foot on unstable surface or equipment. Bodyweight centered over front leg, back leg lifted (no support). Bend down into knee flexion. Keep the torso as erect as possible. Extend front leg and lift free leg backwards.	For intermediate exercisers. Check that both knees are in the right position and aligned with the feet. Focus equally on the concentric and the eccentric phase of the exercise.	Different arm position. With or without movement in the free leg. Use a variety of equipment, for stability work. Here a rolled-up mat is used.

EXERCISE	TECHNIQUE	

**REAR LUNGE
WITH LEG CIRCLE**

Primary muscles:
Quadriceps,
gluteus maximus, hamstrings

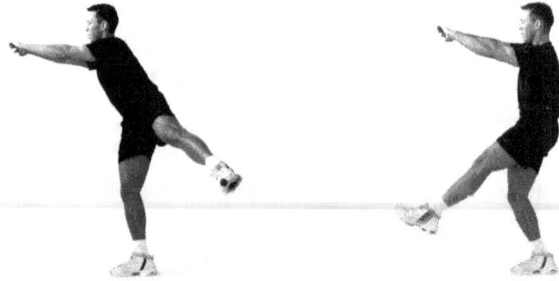

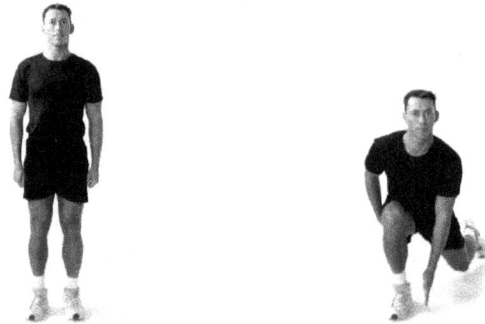

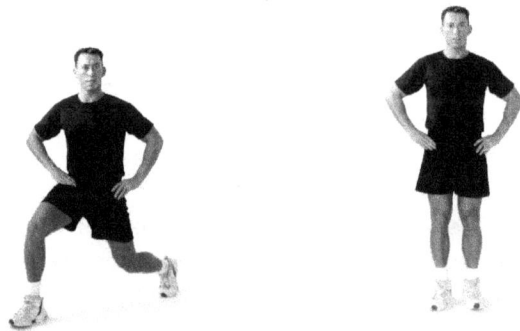

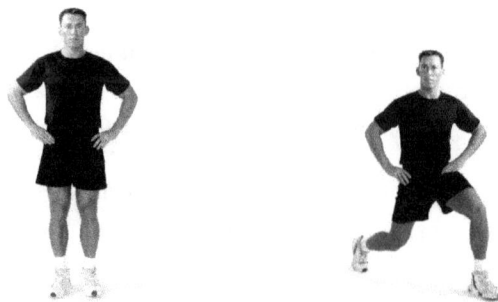

**DIAGONAL LUNGE
HAND-TO-FOOT**

Primary muscles:
Quadriceps,
gluteus maximus, hamstrings

**DIAGONAL LUNGE FRONT
(eg. 45°, between 1 and
2 on imaginary clock)**

Primary muscles:
Quadriceps,
gluteus maximus, hamstrings

**DIAGONAL LUNGE BACK
(REAR DIAGONAL LUNGE)
(eg. 45°, between 4 and 5 on
imaginary clock)**

Primary muscles:
Quadriceps,
gluteus maximus, hamstrings

Standing. Feet hip-width apart. Take a large step backward. Shift weight forward and extend front leg. At the same time make a circle with the back leg, from hip extension, to abduction and flexion, then feet together. Repeat with the opposite or same leg.	Contract the core muscles to stabilize the body. Check that both knees are in the right position and aligned with the feet. Focus equally on concentric and eccentric phase. Requires some hamstring and adductor flexibility.	Different arm exercisex, eg. biceps curl and lateral raise. With or without barbell/ dumbbells/medicine ball.
Standing. Feet hip-width apart. Diagonal lunge 20-45 degrees. Front foot land firmly on floor. Front lower leg vertical. Back foot heel is liftet. Torso slightly forward, touch opposite hand to the inside of the front foot. Push back to starting position. Repeat with the opposite leg.	Contract the core muscles to stabilize the body. Check that both knees are in the right position and aligned with the feet. Focus equally on concentric and eccentric phase. Requires some hamstring and adductor flexibility.	With or without resistance/ medicine ball. Same leg or alternating. **DIAGONAL LUNGE WITH TORSOROTATION** Instead of touching the inside of the foot, turn the torso and touch the outside of the front foot.
Standing. Feet hip-width apart. Diagonal lunge forward. Pivot on back foot as you step. The front lower leg vertical, back lower leg horizontal. Contract buttock and thigh and step back. Repeat with the opposite or same leg. Step in different directions.	For advanced exercisers. Shoulders, torso and hips straight forward. Only the legs turn diagonally. Watch the knees, no twisting. Requires some hamstring and adductor flexibility.	Different arm position. Different angles. With or without barbell/ dumbbells/medicine ball.
Standing. Feet hip-width apart. Lunge diagonally backwards. Pivot on back foot as you step. The front lower leg vertical, back lower leg horizontal. Contract buttock and thigh and step back. Repeat with the opposite or same leg. Step in different directions.	For advanced exercisers. Shoulders, torso and hips straight forward. Only the legs turn diagonally. Watch the knees, no twisting. When stepping backward, look back to check, before first step, that the area is clear. Requires some flexibility.	Different arm position. With or without barbell/ dumbbells/medicine ball.

**MULTI-LUNGE
(MULTI-DIRECTIONAL LUNGE)**

Primary muscles:
Quadriceps,
gluteus maximus, hamstrings

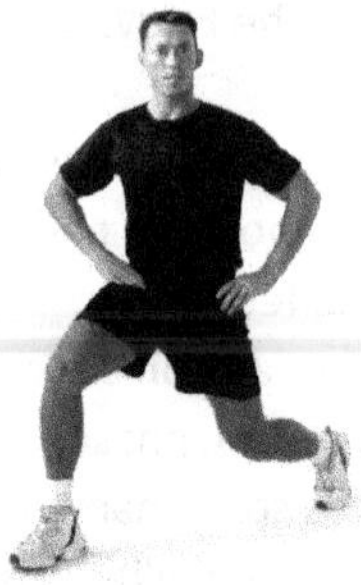

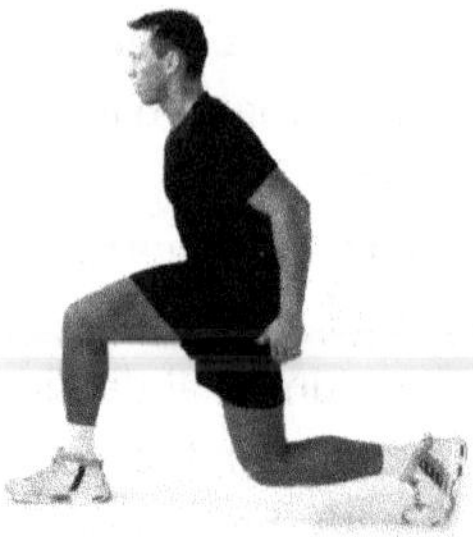

LUNGE JUMP

Primary muscles:
Quadriceps, gluteus maximus,
hamstrings, calf muscles
(soleus and gastrocnemeus)

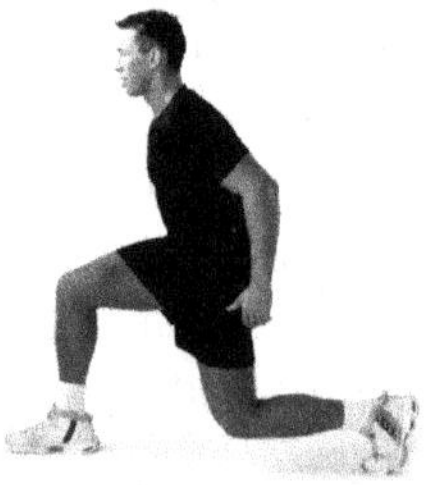

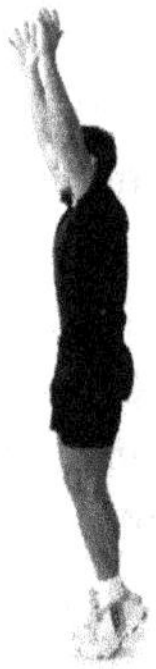

**POWER LUNGE
WITH LEG CHANGE
(JUMPING LUNGE)**

Primary muscles:
Quadriceps,
gluteus maximus, hamstrings

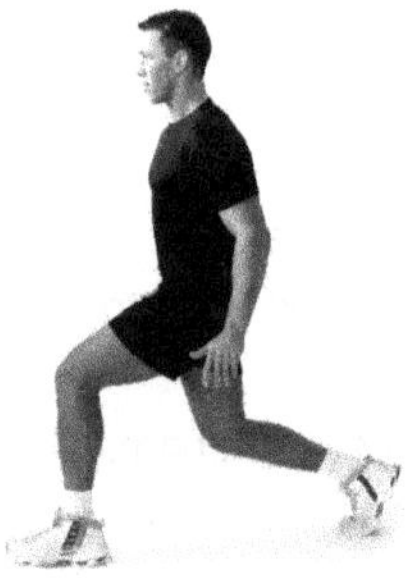

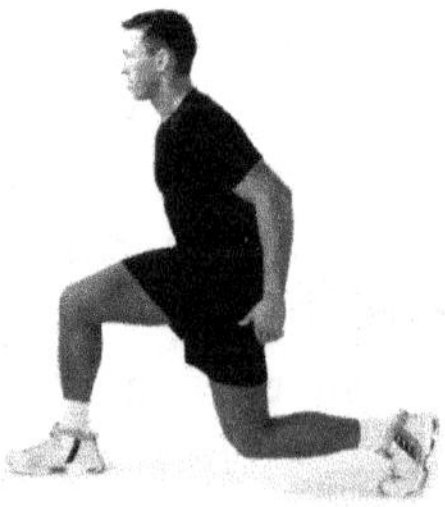

**LUNGE EXTENSION
WITH BENCH AND TUBE**

Primary muscles:
Quadriceps,
gluteus maximus, hamstrings

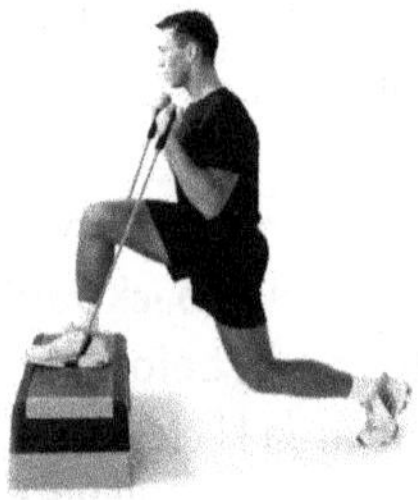

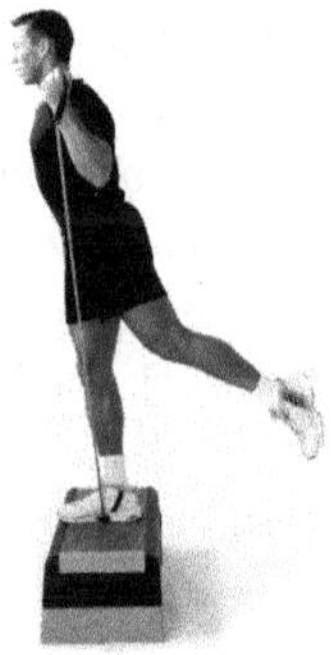

Standing. Feet hip-width apart. A series of lunge steps: Forward, diagonally forward, sideways, diagonally backward, straight backward. Repeat. All directions with one leg at a time – and then the opposite. Or alternate, right and left leg.	For advanced exercisers. Contract the core muscles to stabilize the body. Check that both knees are in the right position and aligned with the feet. Requires some hamstring and adductor flexibility.	With or without resistance. **LUNGE WITH TURN** As a lunge forward, but at the same time pivot on stationary foot turning the body to the side or backward (eg. 90-180 degree turn). When the right foot step, turn right. Be careful not to twist the knee.
Standing. Feet hip-width apart. 1) Lunge forward, 2) step back, feet hip-width apart. 3) Bend the legs slightly and quickly (pre-stretch) and jump as high as you can. 4) Land in the same place. Repeat with opposite leg.	For advanced exercisers. Contract the core muscles to stabilize the body, Check that both knees are in the right position and aligned with the feet. Requires some hamstring and adductor flexibility.	Different arm position. Different leg position. With or without barbell/ dumbbells/medicine ball.
Standing. Feet hip-width apart. Stationary lunge, approx. 90 degr. flexion of both knees). Jump and change legs, so the opposite leg lands in front. Make sure the feet land firmly, all of front foot and ball of back foot, back heel is lifted.	For advanced exercisers. Contract the core muscles to stabilize the body. Check that both knees are in the right position and aligned with the feet. The back heel must be lifted to protect the achilles tendon.	With or without barbell/ dumbbells/medicine ball.
Standing. Feet staggered. Front foot on step, back foot on floor with the heel lifted. Tube or band under front foot. Hold tube with hands on the shoulders. Extend front leg, to lift the body up on the step. Back leg backward in the air. Lower back down carefully, only ball of foot to ground.	Contract the core muscles to stabilize the body. Check that both knees are in the right position and aligned with the feet. Lower back leg carefully to the floor. Control the eccentric phase, land just on ball of foot, protect the achilles tendon.	Bench height may be varied. With tube or band.

**REAR LUNGE
WITH CHEST PRESS
WITH TUBE/BAND**

Primary muscles:
Quadriceps, gluteus maximus,
hamstrings, pectoralis, triceps

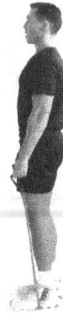

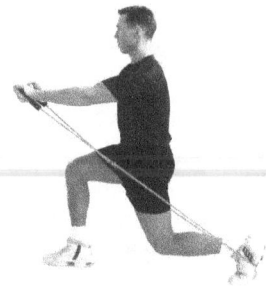

LUNGE WITH KNEE LIFT

Primary muscles:
Quadriceps, iliopsoas,
gluteus maximus, hamstrings

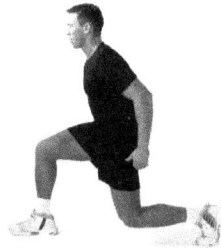

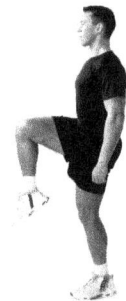

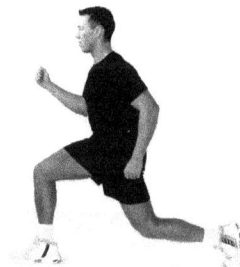

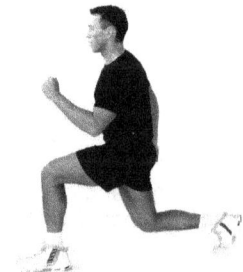

WALKING LUNGES

Primary muscles:
Quadriceps,
gluteus maximus, hamstrings

**SIDE LUNGE STATIONARY,
(SKATER'S LUNGE)**

Primary muscles:
Quadriceps, gluteus maximus,
hamstrings, adductors

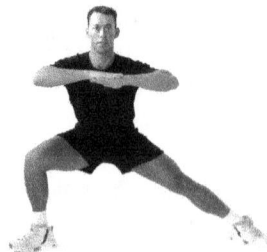

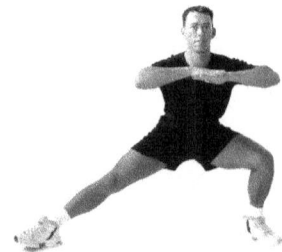

Standing. Legs together. Tube under one foot; step this foot backward in a rear lunge, while the arms press forward in a chest press or front raise. Be careful, so the tube does not slip off the foot. Step forward. Repeat with same leg. After a set, repeat with other foor.	Contract the core muscles to stabilize the body. The core is also worked in this exercise. Check that both knees are in the right position and aligned with the feet. Focus equally on the concentric and the eccentric phase of the exercise.	With tube or band. If you use a resistance band you kan make a loop, binding, around the foot, so the band stays in place. With a tube you must be careful, so the tube does not come off.
Standing. Feet hip-width apart. Contract the core to stabilize. 1) Take a large step forward, from this lunge position 2) lift the front leg up into kneelift 3) back into lunge position, 4) push/step back to starting position. Repeat with the same or opposite leg.	Four phases. For balance work. Check that both knees are in the right position and aligned with the feet. Focus equally on the concentric and the eccentric phase of the exercise. Requires some hamstring and adductor flexibility.	Different arm position. With or without barbell/ dumbbells/medicine ball.
Standing. Take a large step forward (bigger than normal walking steps). Land firmly with all of the foot on the ground. Stabilize and continue going forward with another step. Keep the torso erect and the head lliftet, looking forward (the neck in neutral).	Requires ample space for travelling forward. Check that both knees are in the right position and aligned with the feet. Focus equally on concentric and eccentric phase. Requires some hamstring and adductor flexibility.	Different arm position. With or without resistance. You can step together for every step or continue directly into a new step forward with the opposite foot.
Standing. Very wide stance. Feet parallel or slightly out. Legs bent, close to sumo squat position. Lunge to one side and lunge to the opposite side. The movement is smooth and controlled. The head/torso remains at the same level throughout the exercise.	Contracte the buttocks, gluteus maximus, to pull (rotate) legs backward, so the knees do not rotate inwards. The knees should be aligned with the feet. Contract the pelvic floor muscles.	Different arm position. Add a small pause on each side, in the end ranges of the exercise.

EXERCISE	TECHNIQUE

SIDELUNGE

Primary muscles:
Quadriceps,
gluteus maximus, hamstrings,
abductors andadductors

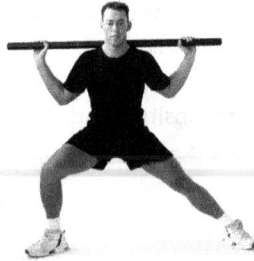

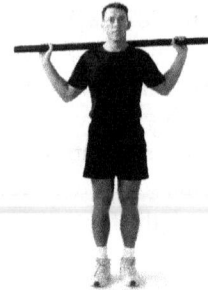

**LUNGE WITH PIVOT
(TRANSVERSE LUNGE)**

Primary muscles:
Quadriceps,
gluteus maximus, hamstrings

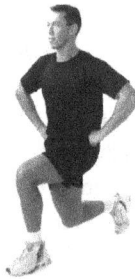

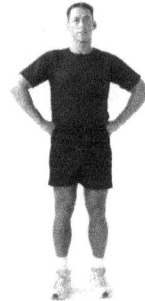

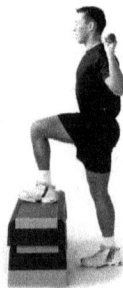

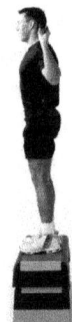

**LUNGE WITH
TORSO ROTATION**

Primary muscles:
Quadriceps,
gluteus maximus, hamstrings,
obliques internus and externus

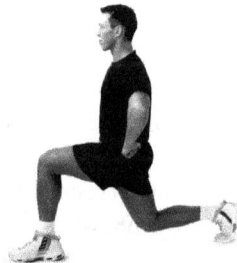

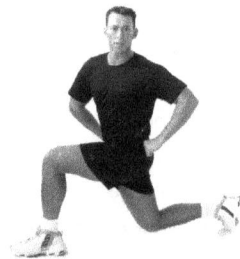

STEP UP

Primary muscles:
Quadriceps,
gluteus maximus, hamstrings

Standing. Feet hip-width apart. Take a large step to one side, with natural outward rotation of the hip. Land with the foot firmly on the floor, lower leg vertical. Contract buttocks and thigh and push off, step back to starting position. Repeat with opposite leg.	Contract the core muscles to stabilize the body. Check that both knees are in the right position and aligned with the feet. Focus equally on the concentric and the eccentric phase of the exercise.	Different arm/leg position. With or without resistance. **SIDELUNGE WITH SIDELIFT** Lunge to the side, from here abduct the outer leg up and out. Leg can lower back into sidelunge before returning back to starting position, or return straight back.
Standing. Feet hip-width apart. One leg step in front of the other, pivot on back foot. Land with front foot firmly on the floor. You pivot by lifting the heel and turning on the ball of the foot. Return the same way back, by reverse pivot.	For advanced exercisers. Recommended for sports training. Important to lift the heel on the pivoting foot, to avoid twisting the knee.	Step out in different directions, eg. from 10 degrees forward and up to a 180 degree turn. **CROSS BODY LUNGE** Step past the midline of the body, past the opposite leg. Torso facing forward, leg, knee and foot diagonal.
Standing. Feet hip-width apart. 1) Take a large step forward. Front foot land firmly on the floor. Front lower leg vertical, back lower leg horizontal. 2) Hold the position, rotate the torso to the side (towards the front leg), 3) rotate back, 4) step back again. Repeat with the opposite leg.	For intermediate to advanced exercisers. Four phases. Can be performed one step at a time in a moderate tempo or as one continuus movement in a faster tempo (for advanced exercisers). Watch the knee: Rotate the torso, not the knee.	Different arm position. With or without resistance/ bodybar (not recommended if you have back- or shoulder-problems).
Standing close to the bench (within a foot's distance). 1) Step up with one foot, extend the knee to lift the body up and 2) step up with the other foot. 3) Step back down with the first foot and 4) down with the second foot. Repeat with the same or opposite leg.	Benchheight may vary – a high bench is for advanced exercisers. Note: Step all the way up with both feet, avoid that either heel hangs over the edge of the bench. Note: Beware of sloppy (common) technique, which may cause injuries.	With or without resistance. **CROSS BOX STEP (advanced)** Stand by the corner of a bench. Step up with the outside leg in front of the opposite leg. Step up with the other leg. Step down with the first leg, behind the opposite leg to the opposite corner. Repeat back.

EXERCISE	TECHNIQUE

STEP UP, SIDEWAYS

Primary muscles:
Hamstrings, gluteus maximus
andquadriceps

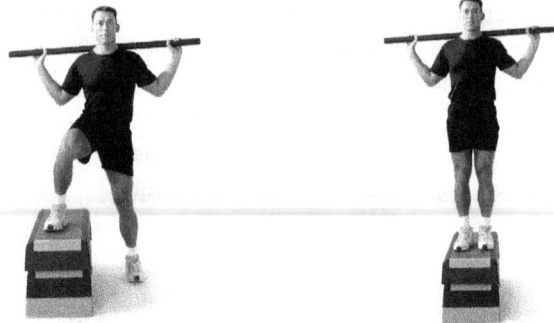

**ONE-LEG SQUAT
(ONE-LEGGED SQUAT)**

Primary muscles:
Quadriceps,
gluteus maximus, hamstrings

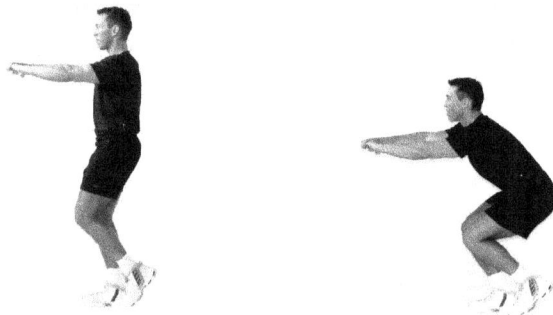

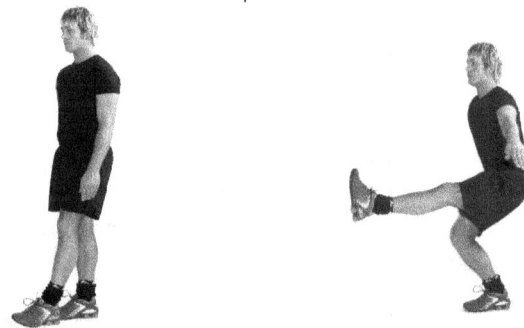

**ONE-LEG SQUAT BALANCE
(PISTOLS, STORK PRESS)**

Primary muscles:
Quadriceps,
gluteus maximus, hamstrings

ONE-LEGGED REACH

Primary muscles:
Quadriceps,
gluteus maximus, hamstrings,
erector spinae

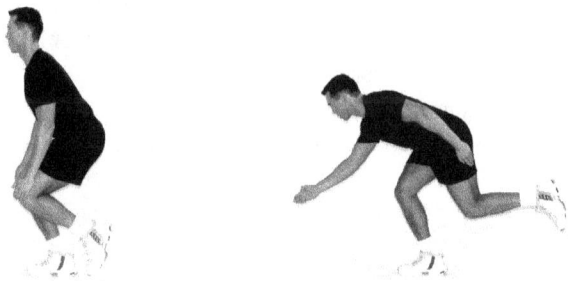

Standing by the side of the bench. 1) Step up with the foot closest to the bench – step all the way up and leave room for the opposite foot – extend leg and 2) step up with opposite leg. 3) Step back down to the starting position, with the last foot up, 4) step down with the first foot up. Repeat.	Benchheight may vary – a high bench is for advanced exercisers. Note: Step all the way up with both feet, avoid that either heel hangs over the edge of the bench. Note: Beware of sloppy (common) technique, which may cause injuries.	Different benchheight. Different arm position. With or without resistance. **STEP OVER THE TOP** You can alternate between right and left by stepping up and the stepping down on the opposite side of the step. Repeat back.
Standing on one leg. Foot firmly on the floor. Opposite leg slightly bent and in front of the other leg (optional position). Torso erect. Look forward. Bend the knee – to a half squat or as deep as possible. Extend knee, go back up.	Keep the foot firmly on the ground. Do not lift the heel during the exercise. Good for balance work. Recommended for sports training.	Different arm position. With or without barbell/dumbbell/ball. With or without support.
Standing on one leg. Foot firmly on the floor. The free leg is straight and lifted (hip flexed) in front of the body. If possible parallel with the floor (throughout exercise). Bend the knee – to a half squat or as deep down as possible. Extend knee, go back up.	For advanced exercisers. Without support the exercise is a super balance exercise. Keep the foot firmly on the ground. Do not lift the heel during the exercise. Requires some hamstring flexibility.	Different arm position. With or without barbell/dumbbell/ball. May be performed with support from a barbell, wall bar or partner.
Standing on one leg. Foot firmly on the floor. The free leg is slightly bent and to the back. Bend the knee and from here lean forward with the torso. The movement upwards is a compound movement: Extend the knee and at the same time return the torso to upright position.	Compound exercise with balance work. Foot firmly on the ground. Do not lift the heel during the exercise. Three phases: 1) Bend, 2) lean forward, 3) extend knee and hip at the same time. Contract the core muscles to stabilize the body.	Different arm position. Different torso/leg range of motion. With or without resistance/ball. With or without support.

SQUAT

Primary muscles:
Quadriceps, gluteus maximus,
hamstrings

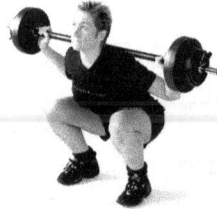

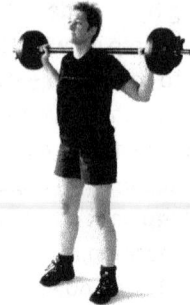

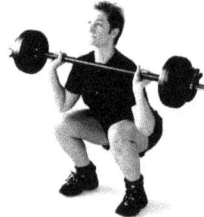

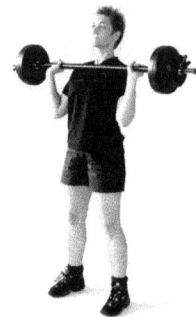

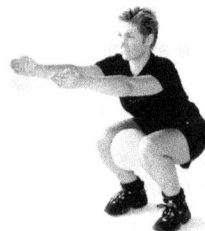

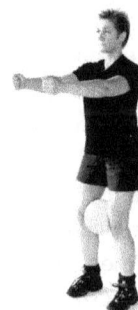

FRONT SQUAT

Primary muscles:
Quadriceps, gluteus maximus,
hamstrings

**SQUAT
WITH ADDUCTION**

Primary muscles:
Quadriceps,
gluteus maximus, hamstrings,
adductors

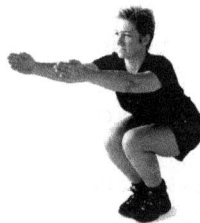

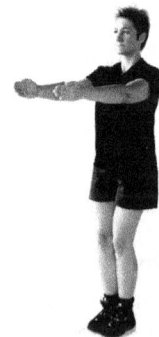

**SQUAT
WITH ADDUCTION
WITH BALL**

Primary muscles:
Quadriceps,
gluteus maximus, hamstrings

TECHNIQUE	ADVICE	VARIATION
Standing. Feet shoulder-width apart. Barbell on upper back and shoulders. Torso erect, look forward. Feet point forward or slightly outward, knees in the same direction. Bend the knees to the desired range of motion. Return to starting position.	Excellent functional exercise. Contract the core muscles to stabilize the body. Torso erect. For fitness do parallel squats (with a heavier load) and – if possible – full squats without weight or a lighter load. Keep knees and feet aligned.	**FULL SQUAT.** Full flexion, for maximal effect, but may be hard on the knees. Advanced. **PARALLEL SQUAT.** Thighs parallel to floor. Traditional. **HALF SQUAT.** Half way ROM. **QUARTER SQUAT.** Small range of motion. Feet together or wide apart. With or without external load.
Standing. Feet shoulder-width apart. Barbell in front of body, top of chest by collarbone. Torso erect, look forward. Feet point forward or slightly outward, knees in the same direction. Bend the knees to the desired range of motion. Return to starting position.	Contract the core muscles to stabilize the body, Torso erect. Keep knees and feet aligned. For fitness do parallel squats (with a heavier load) and – if possible – full squats without weight or a lighter load.	**FULL SQUAT.** Full flexion, for maximal effect, but may be hard on the knees. Advanced. **PARALLEL SQUAT.** Thighs parallel to floor. Traditional. **HALF SQUAT.** Half way ROM. **QUARTER SQUAT.** Small range of motion. Feet together or wide apart. With or without external load.
Standing. Feet together, inner thighs pressing into each other. Torso erect, look forward. Bend the knees to the desired range of motion. Return to starting position.	Contract the core muscles to stabilize the body. Torso erect. Focus on adducting the legs as much as possible throughout the exercise (also end ranges). May be hard on the knees. In this case put a towel or ball between the legs.	**FULL SQUAT.** Full flexion, for maximal effect, but may be hard on the knees. Advanced. **PARALLEL SQUAT.** Thighs parallel to floor. Traditional. **HALF SQUAT.** Half way ROM. **QUARTER SQUAT.** Small range of motion. Feet together or wide apart. With or without external load.
Standing. Feet together. A ball between the legs with Inner thighs pressing against it. Torso erect. Look forward. Feet point forward or slightly outward, knees in the same direction. Bend the knees to the desired range of motion. Keep focusing on adducting. Return to starting position.	This exercise is used in rehabilitation after adductor injuries. Also for variation in group strength training classes. Contract the core muscles to stabilize the body. Keep torso erect.	**FULL SQUAT.** Full flexion, for maximal effect, but may be hard on the knees. Advanced. **PARALLEL SQUAT.** Thighs parallel to floor. Traditional. **HALF SQUAT.** Half way ROM. **QUARTER SQUAT.** Small range of motion. Tiny or small ball. With or without exernal load.

EXERCISE	TECHNIQUE

**ONE-LEG SQUAT
WITH SUPPORT (FOOT)**

Primary muscles:
Quadriceps,
gluteus maximus, hamstrings

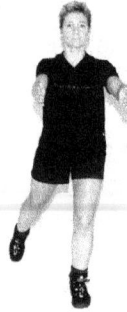

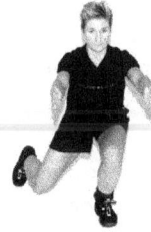

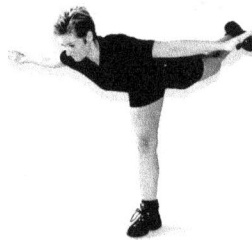

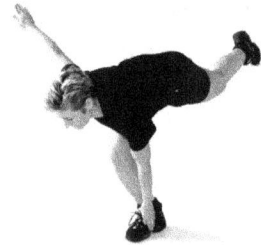

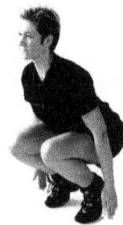

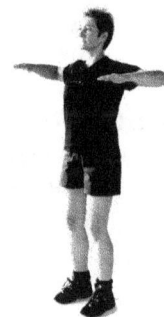

**ONE-LEG SQUAT
IN T-BALANCE**

Primary muscles:
Quadriceps, gluteus maximus,
hamstrings

**ONE-LEG SQUAT
IN T-BALANCE
WITH TORSOROTATION**

Primary muscles:
Quadriceps, gluteus maximus,
hamstrings, obliques

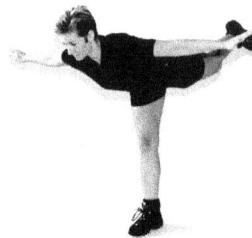

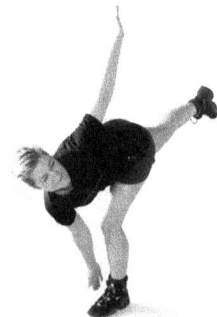

HINDU SQUAT

Primary muscles:
Quadriceps,
gluteus maximus, hamstrings

Standing on one leg. Foot firmly on the floor. The other leg extended back with the toe down for support. Bodyweight is forward, over the front leg. Bend the front knee. Extend the knee, return back up. Repeat.	Hold front foot firmly on the ground. Do not lift the heel during the exercise. Keep knee and foot aligned. Keep the bodyweight forward, do not shift weight back. Back leg support is just for balance.	Different arm position.
Standing on one leg. Foot firmly on the floor. Torso forward in a T-balance, free leg in horizontal. Bend the knee, squat, and touch opposite hand to the inside of the ankle. Go back up. Bend the knee and touch same side hand to the outside of the ankle. Go back up. Repeat.	Excellent for balance work. Keep the foot firmly on the ground. Do not lift the heel during the exercise. Knee and foot aligned, pointing the same way. Contract all muscles on the back of the body, this makes balancing easier.	Different arm position.
Standing on et leg. Foot firmly on the floor. Torso forward in a T-balance, free leg in horizontal. Bend the knee and rotate the torso to one side. Go back up. Bend the knee and rotate the torso to the other side. Repeat.	Excellent for balance work. Keep the foot firmly on the ground. Do not lift the heel during the exercise. Knee and foot aligned, pointing the same way. Contract all muscles on the back of the body, this makes balancing easier.	Different arm position.
Standing. Feet shoulder-width apart. Bend the knees, pull the arms backward. When legs are bent, lift the heels and pull the arms forward with the fingers touching the floor. Extend the knees, go back up, and lift the arms forward/up. In top position, lower the heels and pull arms back. Repeat.	For intermediate to advanced exercisers.Super exercise for leg work and balance. Arms move in a circular flowing motion. Note: Pay special attention: The feet and knees must be aligned, point in the same direction, at all times.	Different arm positions/work.

EXERCISE	TECHNIQUE

**ONE-LEG SQUAT
WITH ABDUCTION**

Primary muscles:
Quadriceps,
gluteus maximus, hamstrings,
(gluteus medius and minimus)

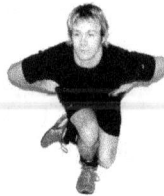

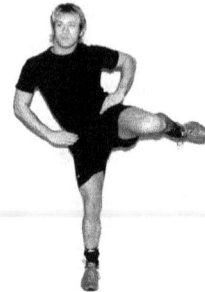

**ONE-LEG SQUAT
WITH HIP ROTATION**

Primary muscles:
Quadriceps,
gluteus maximus, hamstrings

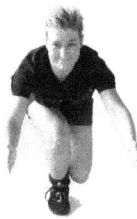

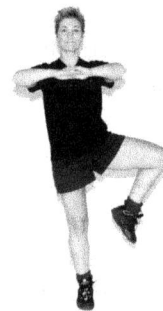

**ONE-LEG SQUAT
WITH HIP ROTATION
AND SIDE BEND**

Primary muscles:
Quadriceps, gluteus maximus,
hamstrings, obliques

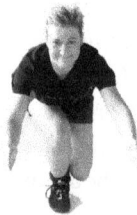

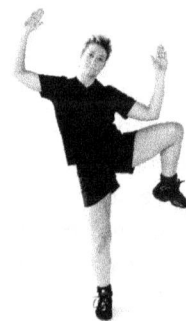

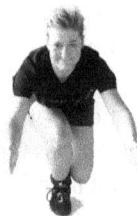

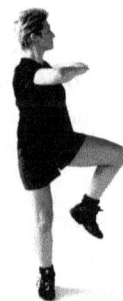

**ONE-LEG SQUAT WITH
TORSO ROTATION**

Primary muscles:
Quadriceps,
gluteus maximus, hamstrings,
obliques

Standing on one leg. Foot firmly on the floor. Free leg is bent. Torso erect. Look forward. Bend the knee, as much as you can. Extend the knee, go up, and lift the free leg (abduct) to the side, to horizontal plane. Or do an outward rotation. Repeat.	For intermediate exercisers. For strength and balance. Keep the foot firmly on the ground. Do not lift the heel during the exercise. Keep knee and foot aligned. Contract the core muscles to stabilize the body.	Different arm position. Different leg exercises in top position. **DEEP ONE-LEG SQUAT** For advanced exercisers. Bend the working leg and touch the free leg knee to the working leg ankle. With or without support.
Standing on one leg. Foot firmly on the floor. Free leg is bent. Torso erect. Look forward. Bend the knee, squat. Extend the knee, go up, and at the same time rotate the free leg outward at the hip. Repeat.	For intermediate exercisers. For strength and balance. Keep the foot firmly on the ground. Do not lift the heel during the exercise. Keep knee and foot aligned. One progression at a time: 1) squat, 2) hip rotation	Different arm position. With or without support.
Standing on one leg. Foot firmly on the floor. Free leg is flexed and liftet. Bend the knee, squat. Extend the knee, go up, and at the same time rotate the free leg outward at the hip. At the end of the movement sidebend the torso to the lifted leg. Repeat.	For intermediate exercisers. For strength and balance. Keep the foot firmly on the ground. Do not lift the heel during the exercise. Keep knee and foot aligned. Contract the core muscles to stabilize the body.	Different arm position.
Standing on one leg. Foot firmly on the floor. Free leg is flexed and liftet. Bend the knee, squat. Extend the knee, go up, and at the same time rotate the free leg outward at the hip. At the end of the movement rotate the torso to the side of the leg. Repeat.	For advanced exercisers. For strength and balance. Keep the foot firmly on the ground. Do not lift the heel during the exercise. Keep knee and foot aligned. Practice one step at a time: 1) squat, 2) hip rotation, 3) torso rotation	Different arm position. With or without support.

EXERCISE	TECHNIQUE

**SQUAT
WITH DUMBBELLS**

Primary muscles:
Quadriceps, gluteus maximus,
hamstrings

ZERCHER SQUAT

Primary muscles:
Quadriceps, gluteus maximus,
hamstrings

OVERHEAD SQUAT

Primary muscles:
Quadriceps, gluteus maximus,
hamstrings, deltoids, triceps

BARBELL HACK SQUAT

Primary muscles:
Quadriceps, gluteus maximus,
hamstrings

Standing. Feet shoulder-width apart. A dumbbell in each hand, the arms at sides. Torso erect. Look forward. Feet forward or slightly outward. Knees in the same direction. Bend the knees to the desired range of motion. Return.	Contract the core muscles to stabilize the body, Control the movement, avoid that the knees rotate inward. Knees and feet aligned. **SQUAT WITH ADDUCTION** Provides variation, but may be har don the knees. Tip: Hold a small ball between the knees.	**FULL SQUAT**. Full flexion, for maximal effect, but may be hard on the knees. Advanced. **PARALLEL SQUAT**. Thighs parallel to floor. Traditional. **HALF SQUAT**. Half way ROM. **QUARTER SQUAT**. Small range of motion. Feet together or wide apart. With or without external load.
Standing. Feet hip or shoulder-width apart. The arms bent, barbell held by the bent arm (at elbow joints). Torso erect. Look forward. Feet forward or slightly out. Knees in the same direction. Bend the knee to desired range of motion. Return.	Contract the core muscles to stabilize the body, Torso erect. Control the movement, avoid that knees rotate inward. Knees and feet must point same way.	**FULL SQUAT**. Full flexion, for maximal effect, but may be hard on the knees. Advanced. **PARALLEL SQUAT**. Thighs parallel to floor. Traditional. **HALF SQUAT**. Half way ROM. **QUARTER SQUAT**. Small range of motion. Feet together or wide apart. With or without external load.
Standing. Feet shoulder-width apart. Feet forward or slightly out. The knees in same direction. The arms raised above the head, elbows straight, locked. Arms are held as vertical as possible during the entire exercise. Torso erect. Bend the knees. Return.	For advanced exercisers. Good exercise for working the posture. Weightlifting exercise. Not recommended for people with back- or shoulder-problems.	**FULL SQUAT**. Full flexion, for maximal effect, but may be hard on the knees. Advanced. **PARALLEL SQUAT**. Thighs parallel to floor. Traditional. **HALF SQUAT**. Half way ROM. **QUARTER SQUAT**. Small range of motion. Feet together or wide apart. With or without external load.
Standing. Feet shoulder-width apart. The hands hold barbell behind the body. Bend the knees, go down into parallel squat. Lead with the hips. Keep torso erect. Extend the knees. Return up.	Contract the core muscles to stabilize the body, Keep torso erect. The exercise may be hard on the knees.	Different distance between feet, narrow or wide stance.

EXERCISE	TECHNIQUE

BOX/BENCH SQUAT

Primary muscles:
Quadriceps,
gluteus maximus, hamstrings

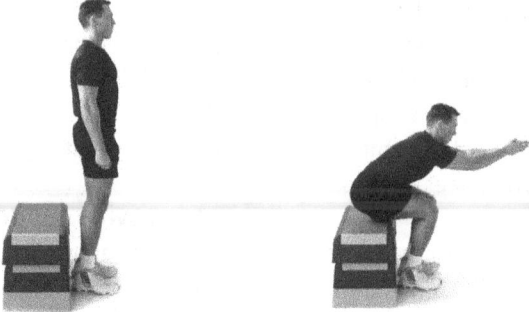

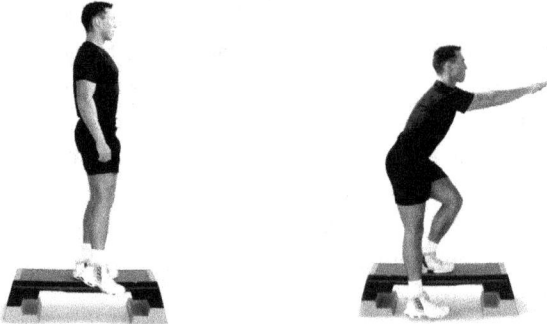

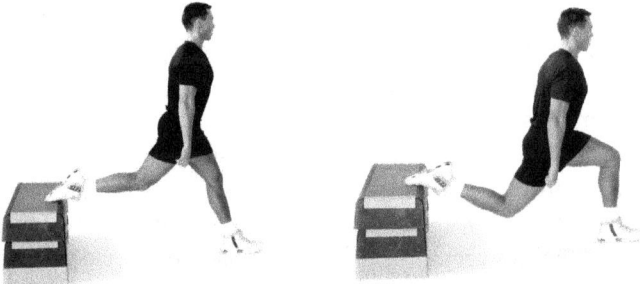

**ONE-LEG DIP
FROM BENCH**

Primary muscles:
Quadriceps,
gluteus maximus, hamstrings

BULGARIAN SQUAT

Primary muscles:
Quadriceps,
gluteus maximus, hamstrings

SISSY SQUAT

Primary muscles:
Quadriceps

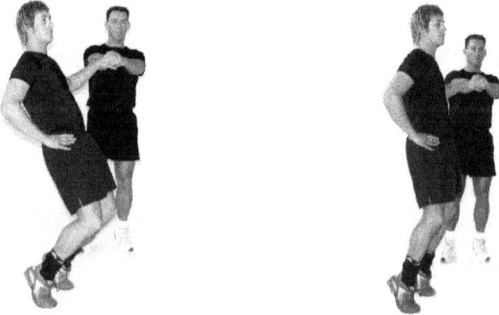

TECHNIQUE	NOTES	VARIATION
Standing. Feet shoulder-width apart. Torso erect. Look forward. Feet forward or slightly out. Knees in the same direction. Bend the knees and touch the bench slightly (40-50 cm high bench). Do not pause. Extend knees, return.	Contract the core muscles to stabilize the body, Torso erect. Control the movement, avoid that knees rotate inward. Knees and feet must point same way.	Different arm position. Different leg position. Different benchheight. With or without resistance. **SQUAT FROM THE TOP** Stand on the top, parallel squat down to the floor with one leg. Repeat with same or opposite leg.
Standing on the top of bench. Working leg is on the bench with foot firmly on the bench. Free leg is by the side of the edge. Bend the knee of the working leg and lower the free leg down, until the foot is just above the floor (or touches it). Extend the knee, return.	Contract the core muscles to stabilize the body. Torso erect, look forward. The exercise may be hard on the knees. Good for balance work.	Different arm position. With or without resistances/barbell. Different bench height, from approx. 20-60 cm. At a higher benchheight you may perform deep squats.
Standing. Back to the bench. Feet staggered. Front foot firmly on the floor. Back leg slightly bent, relaxed, and foot resting on top of a bench, approx. 50-60 cm high. Bend the front knee, go down to half or parallel squat. Extend knee, return up.	Start with the weaker leg. Train one leg at a time, as it difficult to alternate the legs, getting in and out of the position. Good for balance work.	Different benchheight. Different arm position. Different leg position. With or without barbell/ dumbbells/ball. With back foot on a ball, BOSU or teeter board.
Standing. Feet shoulder-width apart. Support from partner or wall bar. Lean the body backwards. The knees go forward, bend the knees, heels are lifting. Go back up again. Focus on using the quadriceps (thigh). No hip movement during the exercise.	Focus on quadriceps. The movement is in the knees. Contract the core muscles to stabilize the body. The exercise may be hard on the knees. Provide some balance work.	Different range of motion.

EXERCISE	TECHNIQUE

**WALL SIT
(WALL SQUAT)**

Primary muscles:
Quadriceps, gluteus maximus

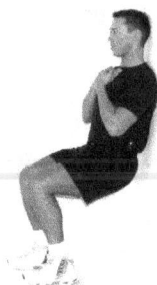

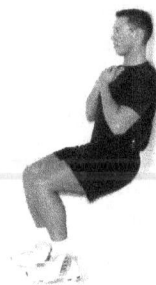

**SQUAT, WIDE STANCE
(PLIE SQUAT, SUMO SQUAT)**

Primary muscles:
Quadriceps, gluteus maximus,
hamstrings, adductors

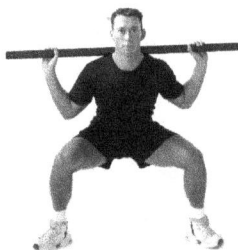

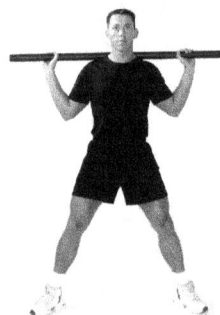

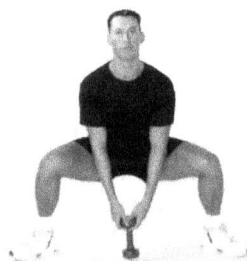

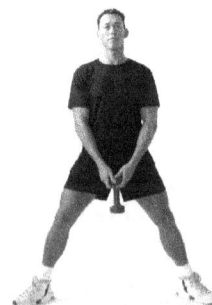

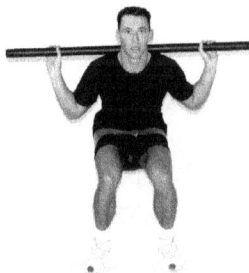

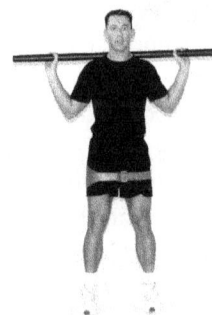

JEFFERSON SQUAT

Primary muscles:
Quadriceps, gluteus maximus,
hamstrings, adductors

BELT SQUAT

Primary muscles:
Quadriceps, gluteus maximus,
hamstrings

Sitting in parallel squat. Feet firmly on the floor. Arm position is optional. The back is supported on wall, wall bar or partner. Hold the position isometrically for as long as desired.	Watch the legs. Avoid that knees rotate inward. Knees and feet must be aligned. Remember to keep breathing. Often used as an exercise in basic training for alpine skiing.	Different arm position. Different leg position. Supported or unsupported.
Standing. Feet wide apart. Barbell on the upper back and the shoulders. Torso erect. Look forward. Feet outward, the knees ind the same direction. Bend the knees in the desired range of motion. Extend the knees, return up.	Contract the core muscles to stabilize the body. Contract the pelvic floor. Contract the buttocks to keep the thighs outward, avoid that knees rotate inward. Knees and feet must be aligned.	With or without barbell/ dumbbells/ball. Note: Different sources mention different starting positions, how wide the feet should be apart, for the sumo squat position.
Standing. Feet wide apart. The arms down in front of the body with the dumbbell in the hands. Torso erect. Look straight forward. Feet out, knees in the same direction. Bend the knees, until thighs are at horizontal level and the dumbbell touches floor. Extend the knees, return up.	Contract the core muscles to stabilize the body. Contract the pelvic floor. Torso erect, look forward. Contract the buttocks to keep the thighs outward, avoid that knees rotate inward. Knees and feet must be aligned.	With or without dumbbell/medicine ball.
Standing. Feet shoulder-width apart. Weightlifting belt around thighs. Torso erect, look straight ahead. Feet forward or slightly outward. The knees in the same direction. Bend the knees, into desired range of motion. Extend the knees, return up.	Technique exercise. For learning to keep the knees aligned with the feet. Feedback: If the belt falls down to the feet, it is because the thighs, knees, has moved inwards.	Different leg position. With or without dumbbell/barbell/ball.

EXERCISE	TECHNIQUE

**SQUAT
WITH TUBE OR BAND**

Primary muscles:
Quadriceps, gluteus maximus,
hamstrings, adductors

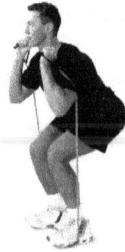

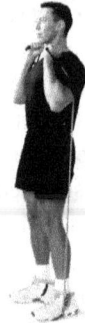

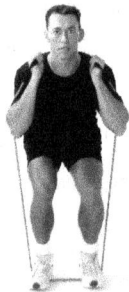

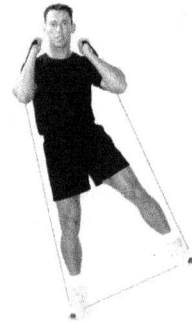

**SQUAT WITH ABDUCTION
WITH TUBE**

Primary muscles:
Quadriceps, gluteus maximus,
hamstrings

**ONE-LEG PRESS
WITH FRONT RAISE
STANDING WITH BAND**

Primary muscles:
Gluteus maximus, hamstrings,
quadriceps, transversus
abdominis, deltoids

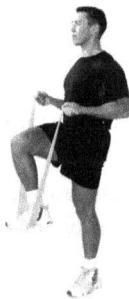

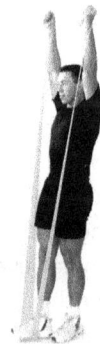

**ONE-LEG PRESS WITH
ONE-ARM FRONTRAISE
SIDELYING WITH BAND**

Primary muscles:
Quadriceps, gluteus maximus,
hamstrings, deltoids

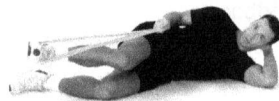

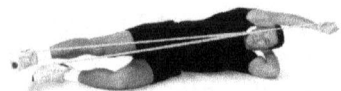

TECHNIQUE	INSTRUCTIONS	VARIATION
Standing. Feet hip- or shoulder-width apart. Tube under feet and held by the hands by the shoulders. Torso erect. Look forward. Bend the knees to the desired range of motion. Extend the knees, return up.	Contract the core muscles to stabilize the body. Control the movement, avoid that knees rotate inward. Knees and feet must be aligned.	Vary distance between feet. Range of motion small or large: Quarter or half or parallel squat. With tube or band.
Standing. Feet shoulder-width apart. Tube under the feet and held anchored at shoulders. Torso erect. Look forward. Bend the knees to the desired range of motion. Extend the knees and at the same time lift one leg to the side, abduct, against the resistance. Lower, go straight into next squat.	Contract the core muscles to stabilize the body. Control the movement, avoid that knees rotate inward. Knees and feet must be aligned.	Vary distance between feet. Range of motion small or large: Quarter or half or parallel squat. With tube or band. Alternate between left and right or repeat on same leg.
Standing on one leg. Band around foot on the working leg. Leg is liftet, 90 degree hip flexion. Band in the hands. Arms bent, close to the side of the torso. Extend the working leg, 'step down', while arms lift into a high front raise. Foot on the working leg stops just above the floor. Repeat.	Contract the core muscles to stabilize the body. Works the balance.	Different arm position. Different leg position.
Sidelying. Band around the top foot. Band held by top hand. Leg starts in 90 degree hip flexion. Extend working leg in line with the torso, just above bottom leg. At the same time the top arm lifts into a high front raise. Return.	Contract the core muscles to stabilize the body. Resist the movement, control the eccentric phase of the movement. Note: The lower leg may be bent (easier for keeping the balance) or straight.	Different arm movement.

EXERCISE	TECHNIQUE

**LEG PRESS/FRONT RAISE
ALTERNATING
SUPINE WITH BAND**

Primary muscles:
Quadriceps, gluteus maximus,
hamstrings, adductors,
deltoids

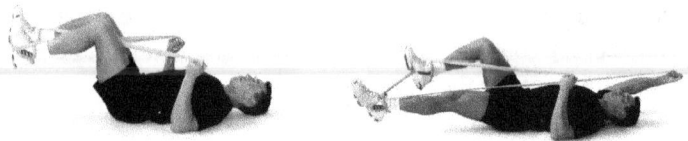

HIP FLEXION, STANDING

Primary muscles:
Iliopsoas, rectus femoris,
tensor fascia latae

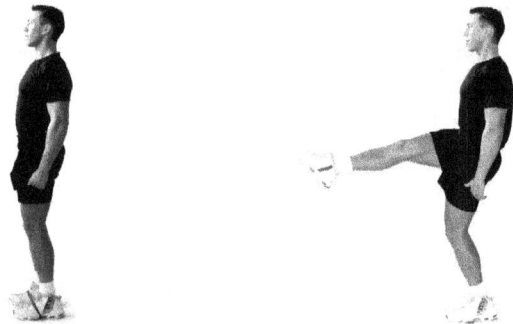

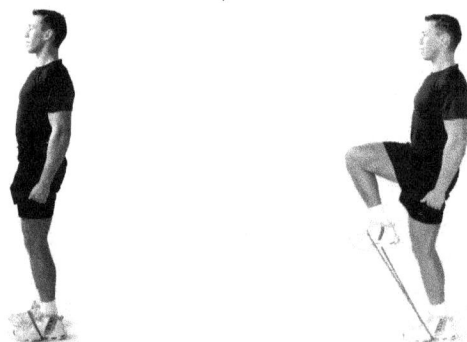

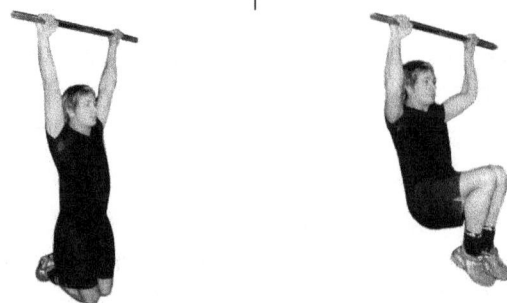

**HIP FLEXION, STANDING WITH
ELASTIC RESISTANCE**

Primary muscles:
Iliopsoas, rectus femoris,
tensor fascia latae

**HIP FLEXION,
HANGING**

Primary muscles:
Iliopsoas, rectus femoris,
tensor fascia latae

Supine. Band under both feet and crossed in front of the legs. The arms are bent, 90 degrees, upper arms at sides. The hands hold each end of the band. Right leg extends, left arm lifts up into shoulder press (or rotation). Lower. Repeat with opposite side.	Contract the core muscles to stabilize the body, avoid over-arching the lower back. Resist the return movement, control the eccentric phase.	Different arm exercises.
Standing. Contract the core muscles to stabilize the body Lift one leg, hip flexion, as high as possible. Hold the position or lower. Lower leg with control.	For strength and balance. Contract the core muscles to stabilize the body. The hip flexor pulls on the lower back, so abdominals must contract to keep the pelvis and spine in neutral, to avoid back problems.	With bent or straight leg. With or without resistance. Isometric or dynamic exercise.
Standing. Rubberband around middle of feet. Lift one leg up, hip flexion. Contract the core muscles to stabilize the body. Lower the leg with control, if possible keep the tension in the rubberband, while continuing.	For balance and strength. Contract the core muscles to stabilize the body. The hip flexor pulls on the lower back, so abdominals must contract to keep the pelvis and spine in neutral, to avoid back problems.	With tube, band or rubberband or ankle weight.
Hanging by the arms. The hands hold onto a wall bar or chin up bar. Contract the pelvic floor. Contract the core muscles. Lift the legs into hip flexion, with knees straight or bent. Contract the abs to lift pelvis and legs. Lower with control. Avoid swinging the body.	For advanced exercisers. Not recommended for people with back problems or weak abdominal muscles. Contract the pelvic floor muscles to withstand the pressure from the abdominal muscles.	With or without resistance. With knees bent or straight.

EXERCISE	TECHNIQUE

HIP FLEXION, SITTING

Primary muscles:
Iliopsoas, rectus femoris,
tensor fascia latae

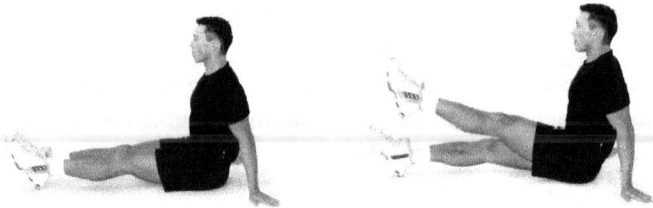

LEG EXTENSION, SITTING

Primary muscles:
Quadriceps, iliopsoas

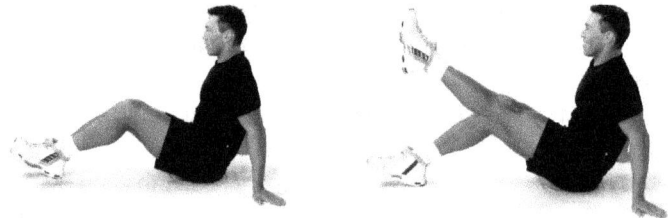

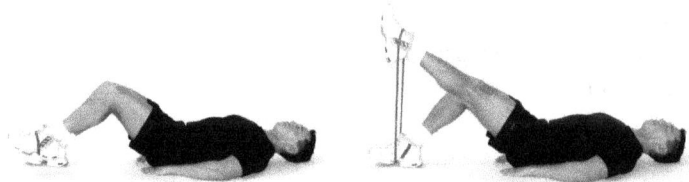

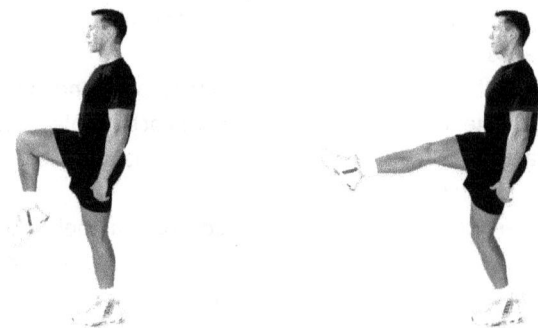

**LEG EXTENSION, SUPINE
WITH RUBBERBAND**

Primary muscles:
Quadriceps, iliopsoas

**LEG EXTENSION, STANDING
(LEG EXTENSION)**

Primary muscles:
Quadriceps, iliopsoas

TECHNIQUE	NOTE	VARIATION
Sitting. Torso erect with hands on he floor or supporting on the forearms. Contract the core muscles to stabilize the torso. One leg rests on the floor, flexed or straight. Working leg is lifted, hip flexion. Lower leg with control.	Contract the core muscles to stabilize the body. The hip flexor pulls on the lower back, so abdominals must contract to keep the pelvis and spine in neutral, to avoid back problems. Basic exercise for gymnastic supports and jumps.	Different body/leg position. With flexed or straight leg. With or without resistance. Perform isometrically or dynamically, slowly or explosively.
Sitting. Torso erect with hands on the floor or supporting on the forearms. Both legs are bent, feet on the floor. The working leg extends. knee extension, Bend the knee and lower the lower leg with control.	Contract the core muscles to stabilize the body.	Stationary leg may be bent or straight. With or without resistance. With rubberband under the foot of the passive leg.
Supine. One leg rests on the floor, flexed or straight. The working leg starts in flexion, contract the thigh and extend the knee. Bend the knee and lower the lower leg with control. With a rubberband: Anchor it under stationary foot and around ankle of working leg.	Contract the core muscles to stabilize the body. You can hold the hands under the buttocks, so the pelvis tilts a little making it easier to keep the lower back down.	With or without resistance. **PRONE LEG EXTENSION** Prone. One leg straight, other flexed. Band around ankle of the working leg and anchored by the hand. Extend the knee, so the lower leg comes closer to the floor. Or with partner resistance.
Standing on one leg. Lift the other leg, hip flexion, thigh in horizontal. Hold. Extend the knee, so the lower leg comes up. Bend the knee and lower the lower leg with control.	Contract the core muscles to stabilize the body. For balance work. The hip flexor pulls on the lower back, so abdominals must contract to keep the pelvis and spine in neutral, to avoid back problems.	With or without resistance.

EXERCISE	TECHNIQUE

**LEGPRESS, SUPINE
WITH TUBE/BAND**

Primary muscles:
Quadriceps,
gluteus maximus

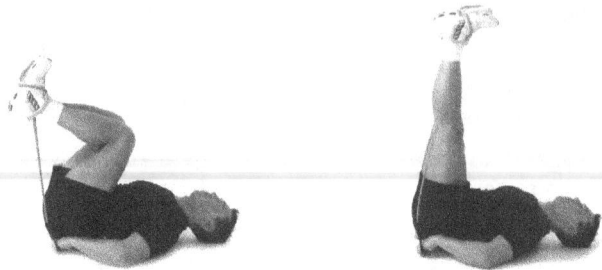

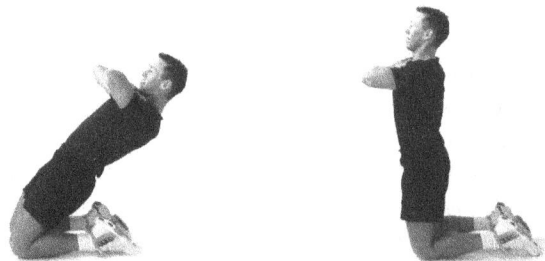

KNEE EXTENSION KNEELING

Primary muscles:
Quadriceps, gluteus maximus

DEADLIFT

Primary muscles:
Erector spinae,
gluteus maximus, hamstrings,
quadriceps, trapezius

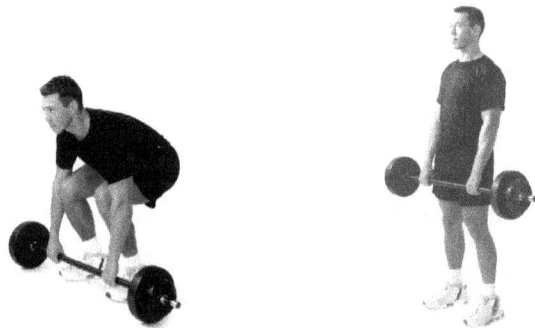

**STRAIGHT LEG DEADLIFT
(STIFF-LEGGED DEADLIFT)**

Primary muscles:
Erector spinae,
hamstrings, gluteus maximus

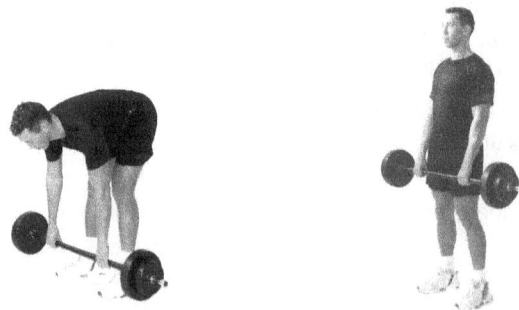

Supine. Tube around feet (use a foot binding). Hands hold the handles under the buttocks. Legs are bent, thighs over the abs. Press the leg upwards, knee and hip extension. Bend the knees, lower the legs with control. Return.	You can hold the hands under the buttocks, so the pelvis tilts a little making it easier to keep the lower back down.	Supine on floor or bench. With tube or band. **LEG EXTENSION** Supine. Same binding. Thighs vertical, lower legs horizontal. Contract thighs and extend the knees, so the lower leg comes to vertical. Lower.
Kneeling. Torso erect. Hips straight. Thighs and abdominal muscles contract. The torso and thighs move backward as one unit. Contract the thighs and lift the body back up to vertical. Repeat.	For advanced exercisers. Not recommended for people with knee problems. Contract the core muscles to stabilize the torso well. Avoid arching the lower back.	Different arm position. With or without dumbbell/medicine ball.
Standing. Feet shoulder-width apart or wider. Legs are bent. The back is straight, torso forward, as erect as possible, look forward. Hold barbell with an overhand grip or combined grip. Lift with the legs and the back. Barbell is kept close to the legs during the entire exercise.	For advanced exercisers. People with back problems needs to lift with perfect technique and pay special attention or avoid deadlift exercises.	Different range of motion and leg position. With dumbbells/medicine ball. **DEADLIFT OFF BOX/** **HIGH DEADLIFT** On a bench or weight plates for greater range of motion. **SUMO DEADLIFT** Feet are wider apart and turned slightly outward.
Standing. Feet hip-width apart. Legs are straight, without hyperextending the knees. The back is straight, torso forward. Look forward. Wide grip with an overhand grip or combined grip. Lift with the legs and the back. Barbell is kept close to the legs during the entire exercise.	For advanced exercisers. Contraindicated exercise. People with back problems needs to lift with perfect technique and pay special attention or avoid deadlift exercises.	Different range of motion and leg position. With dumbbells. **HIGH STIFF LEG DEADLIFT** Stand on bench to increase the range of motion. **SUMO STIFF LEG DEADLIFT** Feet are wider apart and turned slightly outward.

EXERCISE	TECHNIQUE

GOOD MORNING

Primary muscles:
Hamstrings, gluteus maximus,
erector spinae

ROMANIAN DEADLIFT

Primary muscles:
Hamstrings, gluteus maximus

**ROMANIAN DEADLIFT
ONE-LEG/ONE-ARM**

Primary muscles:
Hamstrings, gluteus maximus

**HIP EXTENSION,
STANDING**

Primary muscles:
Gluteus maximus, hamstrings

TECHNIQUE	NOTES	VARIATION
Standing. Feet shoulder-width apart. Legs slightly bent, Keep the back straight. Barbell on the upper back and shoulders. Bend the torso forward, until the body comes close to horizontal position. Lift torso to upright position.	A controversial exercise; hard on the back. Many experts advice against it. Contract the core muscles and kept the back completely straight in all of the exercise. Neck in neutral. Do not 'drop' the head, as this typically results in rounding the back.	With or without resistance. With barbell/dumbbells/ball.
Standing. As a straight-leg deadlift, but start with legs slightly bent. Push the hips back and lower the torso, until it comes close to horizontal position. The barbell is approx. 4-4½ inches, 10-15 cm, from the shins. Return to upright position.	For advanced exercisers. People with back problems should be extra careful or avoid deadlift exercises. Contract the core muscles and kept the back completely straight throughout the exercise.	With or without resistance. With barbell/dumbbells/ball.
Standing on one leg. Other leg is straight and slightly behind stationary leg. Hand on the side of the free leg holds a dumbbell. The torso and leg tips forward into a T-balance, while the dumbbell is lowered straight down. Extend back up with control, moving the hips forward.	Excellent hamstring and balance exercise. Contract the core muscles to stabilize the body. Hips are kept level. Requires some hamstring flexibility.	With or without resistance. **ROMANIAN DEADLIFT WITH MEDICINE BALL OVER HEAD** Stand on one leg, the arms over the head with medicine ball in the hands. Tip all of the body forward in a T-balance. No movement in the arms or legs.
Standing. One leg is extended straight backwards, hip extension (max. 10-20 degrees back). Do not arch the lower back. Lower the leg with control. Keep contracting the gluteus and the hamstrings. Repeat.	Good for balance work and easy hamstring/glute work. Contract the core muscles to stabilize the body. The stationary leg is straight, without hyperextending the knee.	Different arm/leg position. Leg straight or flexed. With or without support. With or without resistance/tube. Different hip movement – eg. 'draw' a triangle or circle to include hip rotation..

EXERCISE	TECHNIQUE

**HIP EXTENSION
STANDING WITH BODYBAR**

Primary muscles:
Gluteus maximus, hamstrings

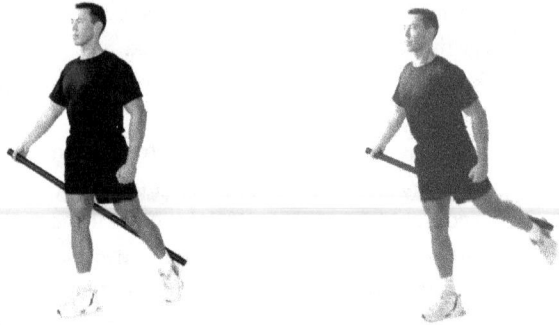

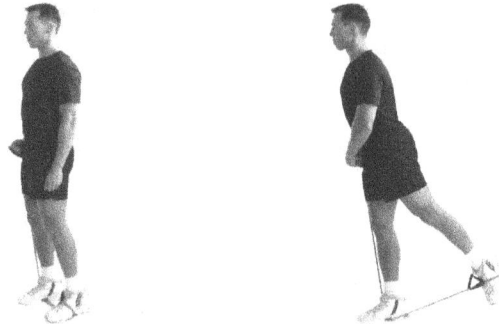

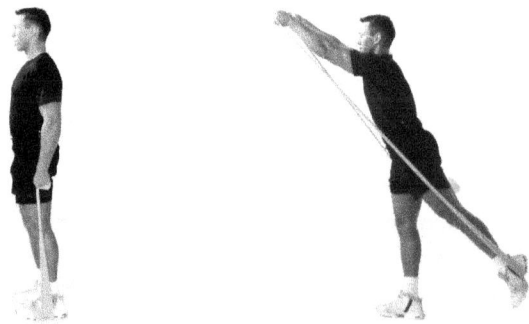

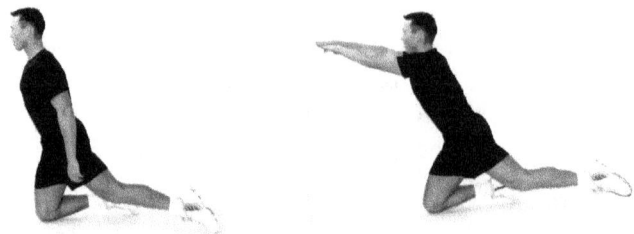

**HIP EXTENSION
STANDING WITH TUBE**

Primary muscles:
Gluteus maximus, hamstrings

**HIP EXTENSION
STANDING WITH BAND/
FRONT RAISE**

Primary muscles:
Gluteus maximus, hamstrings

**HIP EXTENSION
KNEELING**

Primary muscles:
Gluteus maximus, hamstrings

Standing. One foot firmly on the floor. Other leg is extended behind the body. Bodybar rests by the ankle on the back leg. The opposite hand holds the other end of the bodybar. Arm a little to the side. Lift leg up (back) into further extension (approx. 10-20 degrees). Lower with control.	For balance work. The exercise may be difficult to get into, the bodybar rolls off. Avoid arching the back. Contract the core muscles to stabilize the body.	With or without resistance. With or without rotation at the hip.
Standing. Tube looped around foot of the working leg. Opposite foot stands on the tube and the same side hand holds the handle. Extend the leg straight back, hip extension (approx. 10-20 degrees). Avoid arching the lower back. Lower with control.	For balance work. Contract the core muscles to stabilize the body.	With rubberband (around both ankles), with tube or band. You can vary the tube resistance by stepping closer to or away from the working leg.
Standing. Band around foot of working leg. Arms at sides. Hands hold the ends of the band. Extend the leg straight back, hip extension (approx. 10-20 degrees). At the same time lift opposite arm or both arms, front raise. Avoid arching the lower back. Lower with control.	For balance work. Contract the core muscles to stabilize the body. When the band, as shown, is not anchored under opposite foot, the pull on the buttocks and hamstrings is minimal.	With tube or resistance band (with a tube the range of motion is smaller). With band/tube around one foot – or under both feet. Use a foot binding to avoid the tube coming off the foot.
Kneeling on one leg. The other leg is straight back. Lift the back leg straight up into further hip extension. Contract the abdominals to minimize movement of the lower back. Lower with control.	For advanced exercisers. Requires very good flexibility. Limitid range of motion. Basic gymnastic exercise for sagittal split jumps.	With or without support.

EXERCISE	TECHNIQUE

**HIP EXTENSION
PRONE**

Primary muscles:
Gluteus maximus, hamstrings

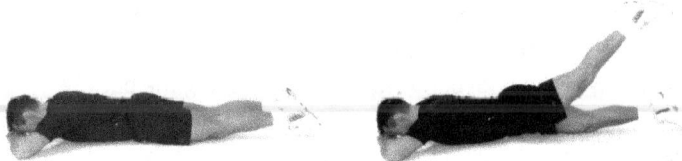

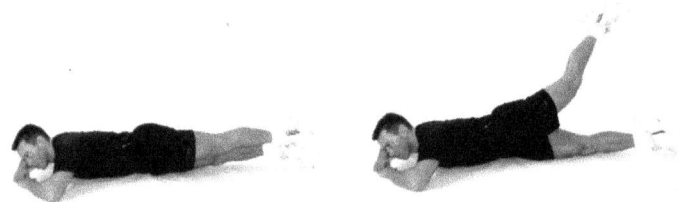

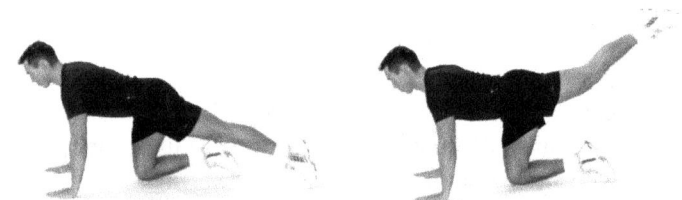

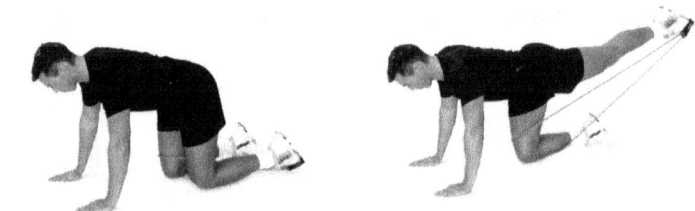

**HIP EXTENSION
HIP TURNED**

Primary muscles:
Gluteus maximus, hamstrings

**HIP EXTENSION
ON ALL FOURS**

Primary muscles:
Gluteus maximus, hamstrings

**LEG PRESS
ON ALL FOURS
WITH TUBE/BAND**

Primary muscles:
Gluteus maximus, hamstrings

Prone. Lift one leg up into hip extension, approx. 10-20 degr. Avoid arching the back. Lower with control. Repeat. After a set repeat with the opposite leg.	Contract the core muscles to stabilize the body. Avoid arching the back.	With straight or flexed leg. With or without ankleweight/ rubberband. On floor, bench or ball.
Prone. A little to one side. Lie on one leg, other leg lifted slightly off the floor. Lift the lifted leg further up into hip extension. Lower with control, stop just before the leg touches the floor. Repeat. After a set repeat with the opposite leg.	Contract the core muscles to stabilize the body. Avoid arching the back.	With straight or flexed leg. With or without ankleweight/ Rubberband. On floor, bench or ball.
On all fours. One leg extended backward, lift it up into extension, approx. 10-20 degrees. Avoid arching the lower back. Lower with control. Repeat. After a set repeat with the opposite leg.	Support on the hands, straight arms, or forearms. When on the forearms, and the body leans forward, working leg must lift higher than horizontal for 10-20 degr. hip extension. Contract the core muscles to stabilize the body. Keep the neck in neutral.	With straight or bent leg. With or without ankleweight. **ON ALL FOURS HIP EXTENSION WITH TUBE** Working leg bent, tube handle around the foot . Tube is anchored by the kneeling leg and the other hand. Lift the leg up against the tube-resistance.
On all fours. Tube or band around foot of working leg. Tube anchored by opposite leg or the hands. The leg starts from a position next to the stationary leg and extends backward into hip extension – approx. 10-20 degrees. Avoid arching the lower back. Lower with control.	Support on the hands, straight arms, or forearms. When on the forearms, and the body leans forward, working leg must lift higher than horizontal for 10-20 degr. hip extension. Contract the core muscles to stabilize the body. Keep the neck in neutral.	With tube or band. Tube-binding: 1) Put both handles around the foot of the working leg, the middle of the tube is anchored by the other leg (by the knee). 2) Put tube under foot , with or without binding, hold both handles with the hands.

EXERCISE	TECHNIQUE

LEGP PRESS
ON ALL FOURS
WITH BAND/FRONT RAISE

Primary muscles:
Gluteus maximus, hamstrings

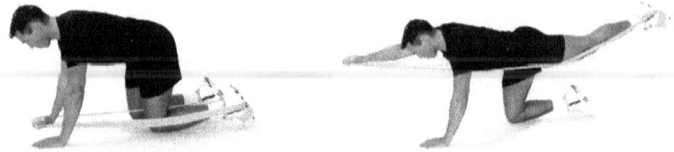

BRIDGE
ISOMETRIC
ONE OR BOTH LEGS

Primary muscles:
Hamstrings, gluteus maximus

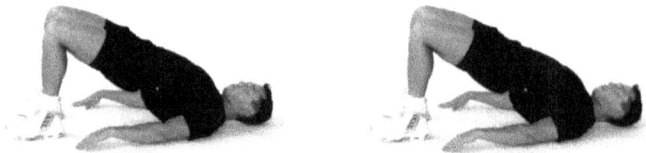

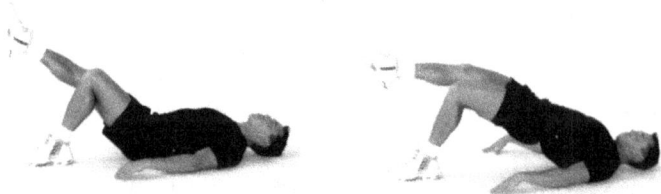

BRIDGE
DYNAMIC
ONE OR BOTH LEGS

Primary muscles:
Hamstrings, gluteus maximus

BRIDGE
WITH ABDUCTION

Primary muscles:
Hamstrings, gluteus maximus
gluteus medius and minimus

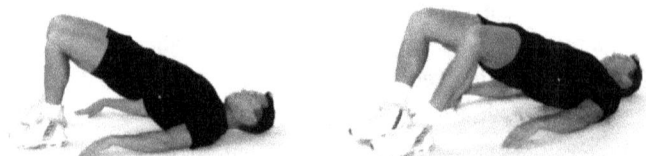

On all fours. Band around foot of the working leg and anchored on the opposite hand. The leg starts from a position next to the stationary leg and extends backward into hip extension – approx. 10-20 degrees. Avoid arching the lower back. Lower with control.	Support on the hands, straight arms, or forearms. When on the forearms, and the body leans forward, working leg must lift higher than horizontal for 10-20 degr. hip extension. Contract the core muscles to stabilize the body. Keep the neck in neutral.	With tube or band.
Supine. Legs bent. Feet hip-width apart on floor, Alternative: Only one foot on the floor with other leg lifted. Contract buttocks and hamstrings and lift the body into bridge position. Support on the shoulders. Hold the position isometrically.	Remember to keep breathing. Contract the buttocks throughout the exercise. Contract the core muscles to stabilize the body.	Different leg position. Unilateral, bilateral. Feet on floor, bench, stability ball or medicine ball.
Supine. Legs bent. Feet hip-width apart on floor. Alternative: Only one foot on the floor with other leg lifted. Contract buttocks and hamstrings and lift the body into bridge position. Support on the shoulders. Lower with control. Repeat.	Keep contracting concentrically and eccentrically – do not rest in the down position. Contract the core muscles to stabilize the body.	Different leg position. Unilateral, bilateral. Feet on floor, bench, stability ball or medicine ball.
Supine. Legs bent. Feet hip-width apart on floor. Contract buttocks and hamstrings and lift the body into bridge position. Support on the shoulders. In bridge position with hips straight, abduct and adduct the legs. Keep hips level. Lower. Repeat.	Remember to keep breathing. Contract the core muscles to stabilize the body. Contract the pelvic floor muscles. Avoid twisting the knees; the feet remain on the floor, but the weight shifts to the outside of the feet.	Different leg position. With or without resistance. Feet on floor, bench, stability ball or medicine ball.

EXERCISE	TECHNIQUE

BRIDGE WALKING

Primary muscles:
Hamstrings, gluteus maximus

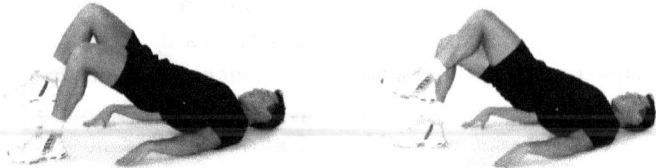

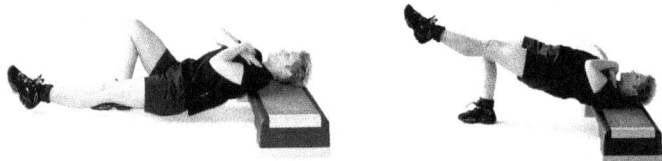

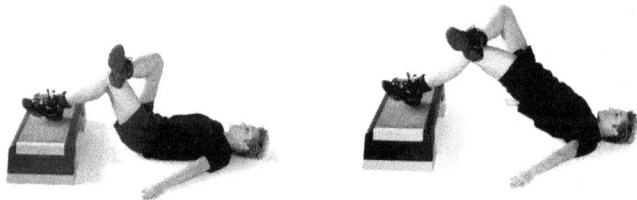

**BRIDGE, ONE LEG,
SUPINE ON BENCH**

Primary muscles:
Hamstrings, gluteus maximus

**BRIDGE, ONE LEG,
SUPINE,
LEG ON BENCH**

Primary muscles:
Hamstrings, gluteus maximus

**EXPLOSIVE HAMSTRING CURL,
PRONE
WITH MEDICINE BALL**

Primary muscles:
Hamstrings

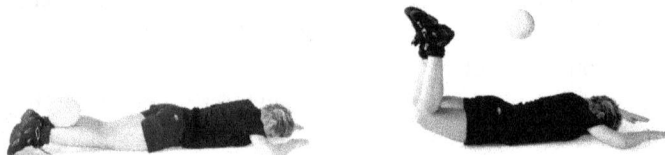

TECHNIQUE	NOTES	VARIATION
Supine. Feet on the floor hip-width apart. Legs bent. Contract buttocks and hamstrings and lift the body into bridge position with support on the shoulders. Hold the position isometrically, while the feet march in place.	Remember to keep breathing. Keep the bridge position throughout the exercise, do not drop the hips. Contract the core muscles to stabilize the body.	Different leg position. Feet on floor, bench, exercise ball or medicine ball.
Supine. Upper back on a bench. One leg bent, foot on the floor, the other leg straight and lifted just above the floor. Contract the buttocks and hamstrings and lift the working leg and hip into bridge position next to the stationary leg. Keep hips level. Lower. Repeat.	Make sure the upper back lies comfortably on the bench. Do not support your bodyweight on the neck. Do not rest in the down position, repeat without pausing.	Bridge position unilateral or bilateral. With bodybar or barbell across the thighs.
Supine. One foot on top of a bench, other leg crossed over, ankle by the knee, thigh out. Contract the buttocks and hamstring and lift the working leg and hip intro bridge position. Lower. Repeat.	Do not rest in the down position, repeat without pausing. Contract the core muscles to stabilize the body.	With bodybar or barbell across the thighs.
Prone. A partner throws a ball onto the lower legs. Bend the legs explosively in order to propel, throw, the ball back to the partner.	The head is kept down. If yo do the exercise without a partner, you have to place and retrieve the ball yourself, more work for you. Contract the core muscles to stabilize the body.	Different balls.

EXERCISE	TECHNIQUE

**HAMSTRING CURL
STANDING**

Primary muscles:
Hamstrings (biceps femoris,
semitendinosus,
semimembranosus)

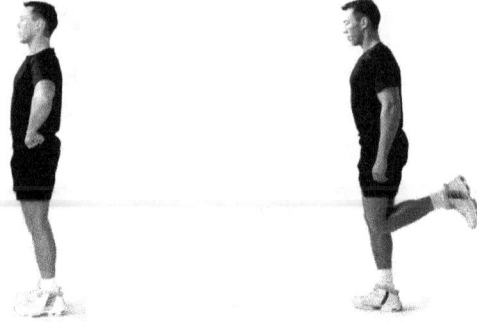

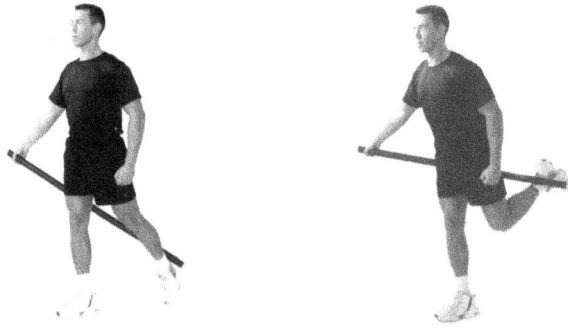

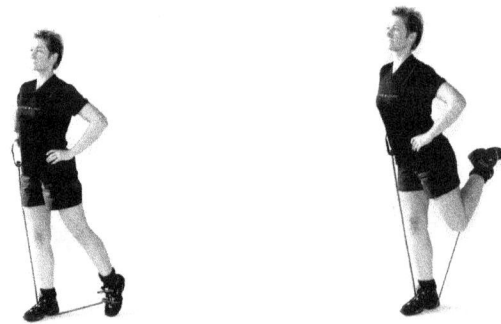

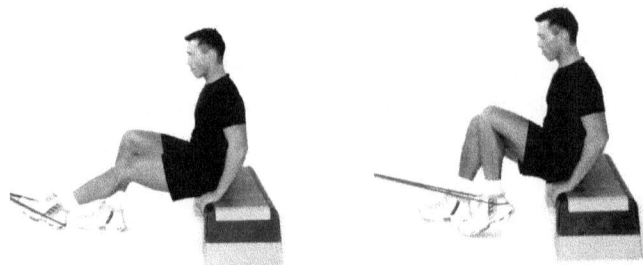

**HAMSTRING CURL
STANDING
WITH BODYBAR**

Primary muscles:
Hamstrings (biceps femoris,
semitendinosus,
semimembranosus)

**HAMSTRING CURL
STANDING
WITH BAND/TUBE**

Primary muscles:
Hamstrings (biceps femoris,
semitendinosus,
semimembranosus)

**HAMSTRING CURL
SITTING
WITH BAND/TUBE**

Primary muscles:
Hamstrings (biceps femoris,
semitendinosus,
semimembranosus)

Standing. Stand on one leg. Bend the other leg, full knee flexion and hip extension, 10-20 degrees. Avoid arching the lower back. Lower the lower leg with control. Repeat.	Minimal strength work without resistance. Some balance work. Contract the core. Relax the lower leg, or plantarflex foot, in order to focus more on the hamstrings than the gastrocnemeus (calf).	With or without resistance, rubberband, tube or band. Rotate leg outward to stress the biceps femoris. Rotate leg inward to stress semitendinosus and semimembranosus.
Standing. Stand on one leg Other leg is extended behind the body. Bodybar on the ankle of the back leg. The opposite hand holds the other end of the bodybar. Arm is a little to the side. Bend the knee as much as Possible, leg above horizontal. Lower with control. Repeat.	Limited range of motion. Contract the core muscles to stabilize the body. Avoid arching the back. Relax the lower leg, or plantarflex foot, in order to focus more on the hamstrings than the gastrocnemeus (calf).	Bodybar support point may vary.
Standing. Stand on one leg. Tube around the foot (a loop). The stationary foot anchors the loop and the hand of the same side hold the handle. Bend the knee as much as possible, lower leg past horizontal. The tube should allow full range of motion. Lower the lower leg. Repeat.	Contract the core muscles to stabilize the body. Make sure that the thigh on the working is behind the stationary leg (hip extension). To keep the tube on the foot, make a loop; put one handle through the other handlle.	With rubberband, tube or band. Rotate leg outward to stress the biceps femoris. Rotate leg inward to stress semitendinosus and semimembranosus.
Sitting on bench. One leg bent with foot on the ground. The other leg straight and lifted well off the ground. Rubberband anchored around a wall bar or bar in front of the body. Rubberband around the ankle of the working leg. Bend the knee as much as possible. Return with control.	Limited range of motion. Contract the core muscles to stabilize the body. After a set repeat with the other leg.	With rubberband, tube or band. Note: With a rubberband range of motion is limited. And with too low a bench range of motion is also limited.

EXERCISE	TECHNIQUE

**LEG LIFT
ON ALL FOURS
WITH DUMBBELL**

Primary muscles:
Gluteus maximus, biceps
femoris, semitendinosus,
semimembranosus

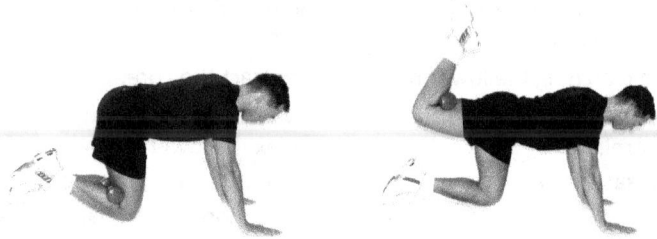

**HAMSTRING CURL
PRONE
WITH RUBBERBAND**

Primary muscles:
Hamstrings (biceps femoris,
semitendinosus,
semimembranosus)

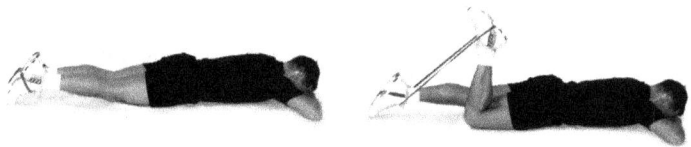

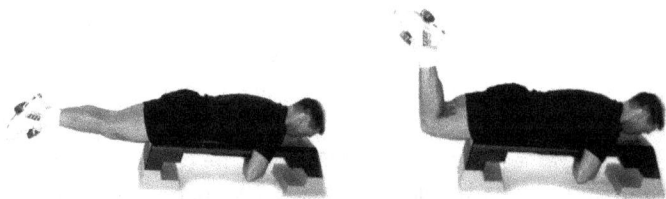

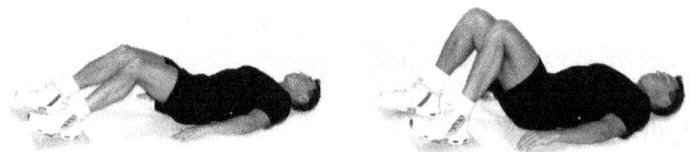

**HAMSTRING CURL
PRONE
WITH DUMBBELL**

Primary muscles:
Hamstrings (biceps femoris,
semitendinosus,
semimembranosus)

**HAMSTRING PULL
SUPINE**

Primary muscles:
Hamstrings (biceps femoris,
semitendinosus,
semimembranosus)

On all fours. The working leg is bent and holds a dumbbell in the hollow of the knee. Lift leg past horizontal into hip extension. At all times contract the hamstrings in order to keep holding the dumbbell. Avoid arching the lower back. Lower with control. Repeat.	Special group resistance training exercise. For variety. Isometric hamstring work with dynamic glute work. Keep contracting the hamstrings. Remember to keep breathing. Contract the core muscles to stabilize the body.	**HAMSTRING PULL'N'CROSS** On all fours with the dumbbell in the hollow of the knee. The working leg is lowered and crossed over past the opposite leg. Lift back up past horizontal.
Prone. Rubberband around both feet. Bend the working leg as much as possible against the resistance. Keep the torso down and avoid lifting the buttocks and arching the lower back. Leg returns with control.	Remember to keep breathing. Contract the core muscles to stabilize the body. Relax the lower leg, or plantarflex the foot, to focus more on the hamstrings than the gastrocnemeus.	Can be performed sidelying for variation. With rubberband, tube, band. Rotate leg outward to stress the biceps femoris. Rotate leg inward to stress semitendinosus and semimembranosus.
Prone. Hold a dumbbell between the feet. Bend the legs until lower legs are almost vertical. Keep the torso down and avoid lifting the buttocs and arching the lower back. Legs are lowered with control.	Remember to keep breathing. Contract the core muscles to stabilize the body. Lower legs stop just before vertical, to keep working against gravity.	On floor or bench.
Supine. Legs slightly bent with feet on the floor, on a piece of carpet, cloth or the like. Press the heels down to create resistance. Bend the legs and pull the feet towards the buttocks. Extend the legs back out, still with the heels pressing down creating resistance.	Remember to keep breathing. Contract the core muscles to stabilize the body.	On floor or bench. Supine or sitting. With medicine ball, stability ball or a piece of cloth or carpet.

EXERCISE	TECHNIQUE

ADDUCTION
SUPINE

Primary muscles:
Adductors

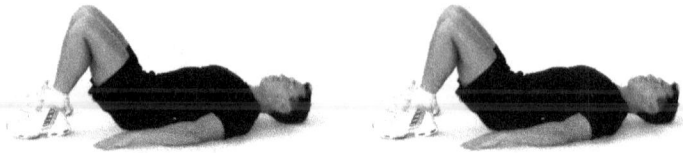

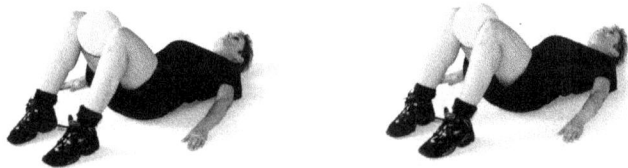

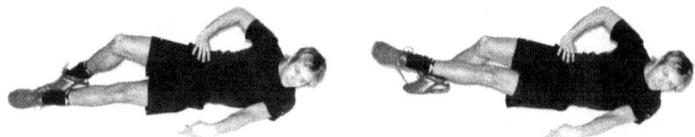

ADDUCTION
BRIDGE POSITION

Primary muscles:
Adductors,
gluteus maximus, hamstrings

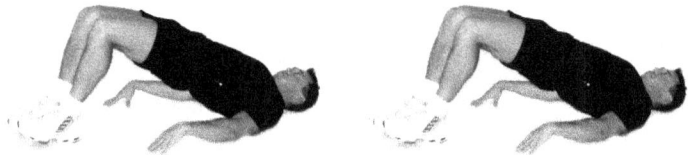

ADDUCTION
SUPINE MED BALL
HIPS AND KNEES BENT

Primary muscles:
Adductors

ADDUCTION
SIDELYING
WORKING LEG STRAIGHT
WITH RUBBERBAND

Primary muscles:
Adductors

Supine. Feet on the floor hip-width apart. Legs are bent. Press thighs together, contract as hard as you can, adduction. Contract isometrically for a few seconds, eg. 5-10 seconds, and release. Repeat.	You can put a towel, a mat or ball between the legs. If legs/knees press directly against each other it may feel uncomfortable. Remember to keep breathing.	Different arm/leg position. Knees bent at different angles. On the floor or legs on a bench.
Supine. Feet on the floor hip-width apart. Legs are bent. Contract the buttocks and hamstrings and lift into bridge position. Hold this position. Press thighs together, contract as hard as possible, adduction. Contract isometrically for a few seconds, eg. 5-10 seconds, and release. Repeat.	You can put a towel, a mat or ball between the legs. If legs/knees press directly against each other it may feel uncomfortable. Remember to keep breathing.	Different arm/leg position. Legs bent at different angles. On the floor or legs on a bench.
Supine. Feet on the floor hip-width apart. Legs are bent and hold a ball between the knees. Press the thighs hard against the ball. Contract isometrically for a few seconds, eg. 5-10 seconds, and release. Repeat.	Remember to keep breathing.	Different arm/leg position. Knees bent at different angles. On the back or in bridge position. On the floor or legs on a bench.
Sidelying. Top leg is bent and behind the opposite leg – with rubberband under the foot and around the ankle of the buttom, working, leg. Adduct and lift the leg off the floor (not just the lower leg). Lower the leg, but do not let it rest on the floor. Repeat.	Keep the torso down, on the floor with the head on the arm, or lift the torso and rest on the forearm. Note: In this position the neck and the shoulders should still be in neutral position. Pelvis and spine in neutral position.	Different body position. The working leg is bent or straight.

EXERCISE	TECHNIQUE

**ADDUCTION
SIDELYING
WITH BODYBAR LIFTED**

Primary muscles:
Adductors

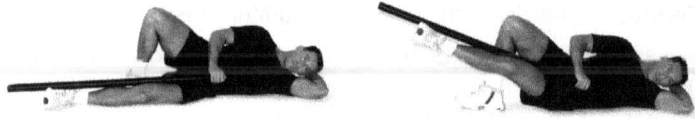

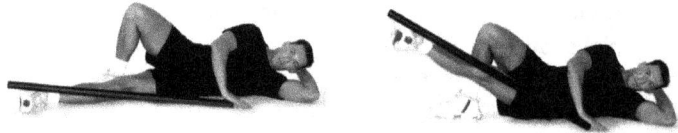

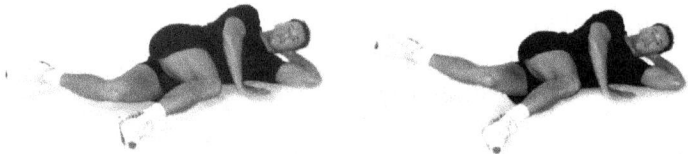

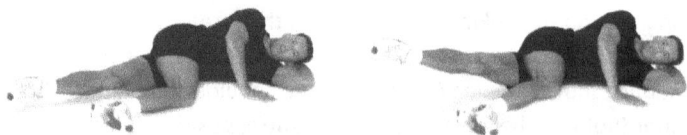

**ADDUCTION
SIDELYING
WITH BODYBAR SUPPORTED**

Primary muscles:
Adductors

**ADDUCTION
SIDELYING
HIP/KNEE BENT**

Primary muscles:
Adductors

**ADDUCTION
SIDELYING
HIP/KNEE STRAIGHT**

Primary muscles:
Adductors

Technique	Notes	Variation
Sidelying. Top leg is bent and behind opposite leg. Bottom leg is slightly bent, so the bodybar rests on three points: Foot, lower leg, thigh. Hold bar steady with the hand (off the floor). Adduct the leg, lift it from the floor. Lower the leg, but without letting go or letting it rest on the floor.	Rest torso on the floor with the head on the arm or the floor. Or lift the torso and rest on the forearm. Note: In this position the neck and the shoulders should still be in neutral position. Keep pelvis and spine in neutral position.	Different leg position, of the top leg, the stationary leg.
Sidelying. Top leg is bent and behind opposite leg. Bottom leg is slightly bent, bodybar rests on three points: Foot, lower leg, thigh. The end of the bar rests on the floor, held steady by the hand. Adduct the leg, lift it from the floor. Lower the leg, but without letting go or letting it rest on the floor.	Rest torso on the floor with the head on the arm or the floor. Or lift the torso and rest on the forearm. Note: In this position the neck and the shoulders should still be in neutral position. Keep pelvis and spine in neutral position.	Different leg position, of the top leg, the stationary leg.
Sidelying. Top leg is kept either in front of or behind the working leg. Bottom leg is slightly flexed with the knee in front of the body and the foot behind it. Adduct the bottom leg, lift it off the floor. Lower the leg, but without resting it on the floor.	Rest torso on the floor with the head on the arm or the floor. Or lift torso and rest on forearm. Note: In this position the neck and the shoulders, pelvis and spine should still be in neutral position. The working leg stays in the same position throughout the exercise.	Different position of top leg: 1. Behind the working leg (WL), leg bent, foot on the floor. 2. In front of the WL, bent leg with foot on the floor. 3. In front of the WL, bent leg with lower leg resting on floor. 4. In front of the WL leg, straight leg forward in front of the body, side of foot on floor.
Sidelying. Top leg either in front of or behind the working leg. Bottom leg is straight and aligned with the torso, no hip flexion. Adduct the bottom leg, lift it off the floor. Lower the leg, but without resting it on the floor.	Rest torso on the floor with the head on the arm or the floor. Or lift the torso and rest on the forearm. Note: In this position the neck and the shoulders should still be in neutral position. Keep pelvis and spine in neutral position.	Different position of top leg: 1. Behind the working leg (WL), leg bent, foot on the floor. 2. In front of the WL, bent leg with foot on the floor. 3. In front of the WL, bent leg with lower leg resting on floor. 4. In front of the WL leg, straight leg forward in front of the body, side of foot on floor.

**ADDUCTION
SIDELYING
HIP/KNEE BENT
WITH RUBBERBAND**

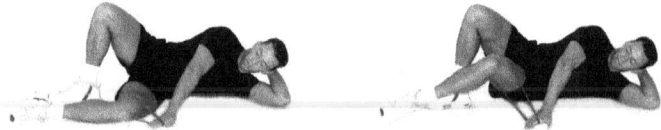

Primary muscles:
Adductors

**ADDUCTION/ABDUCTION
BOTH LEGS LIFTED**

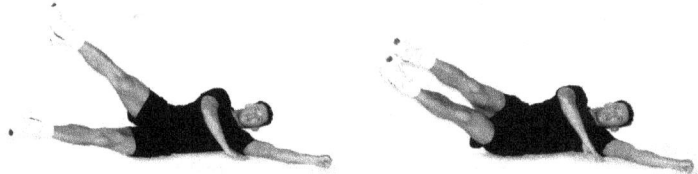

Primary muscles:
Adductors
(abductors, transversus
abdominis).

**ADDUCTION, HIPS FLEXED,
SUPINE WITH TWO
ULTRA-TONERS**

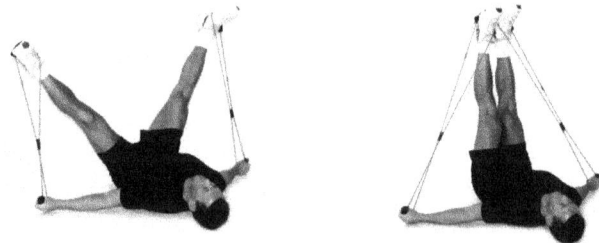

Primary muscles:
Adductors, pectineus,
gracilis, tensor fascia latae

**ADDUCTION, UNILATERAL
WITH A PIECE OF CLOTH**

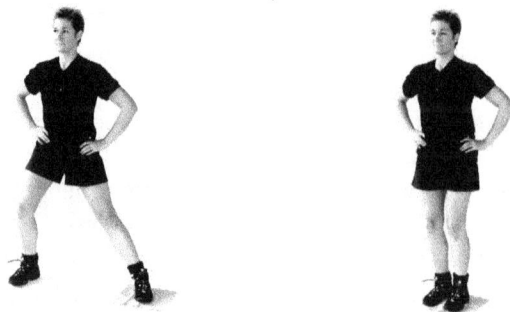

Primary muscles:
Adductors

154

Sidelying. Top leg is bent and behind the bottom leg. Band around the thigh of the working leg and anchored by a hand on the floor. Adduct and rotate leg towards the other leg. The foot stays in contact with the floor. Lower the leg with control.	Rest torso on the floor with the head on the arm or the floor. Or lift the torso and rest on the forearm. Note: In this position the neck and the shoulders should still be in neutral position. Keep pelvis and spine in neutral position.	Different leg position. With rubberband/tube/band.
Sidelying. Both legs are straight and lifted off the floor in frontal plane – top leg directly over the bottom leg. Top leg and bottom leg are abducted and adducted from each other with control.	Rest torso on the floor with the head on the arm or the floor. Or lift the torso and rest on the forearm. Note: In this position the neck and the shoulders should still be in neutral position. Keep pelvis and spine in neutral position.	Different leg position.
Supine. Hip flexed 90 degrees. Legs slightly bent or straight, in vertical and abducted. A large rubberband or 'double-loop' around each foot, anchored by the hands on the floor. The arms are out to the side. Adduct the inner thigh muscles and pull legs together. Return with control.	You can put a towel or mat under the buttocks and small of the back to make it easier to stay in the position. Involves isometric work for the shoulders.	Different arm/leg position. Legs straight or slightly bent.
Standing. One foot firmly on the floor. The other foot is on a piece of cloth and is pushed to the side. Press the foot down to create resistance. Contract the inner thigh muscles and pull, adduct, the working leg towards the stationary leg. Repeat.	The knees face forward. Create resistance by pressing the foot against the piece of cloth or carpet. Note: When using carpet, the carpet pile should be towards the floor, otherwise there is too much resistance, which is uncomfortable for the knee.	With a piece of cloth or carpet.

EXERCISE	TECHNIQUE

**ADDUCTION, UNILATERAL,
STANDING ON SLIDERAMP**

Primary muscles:
Adductors

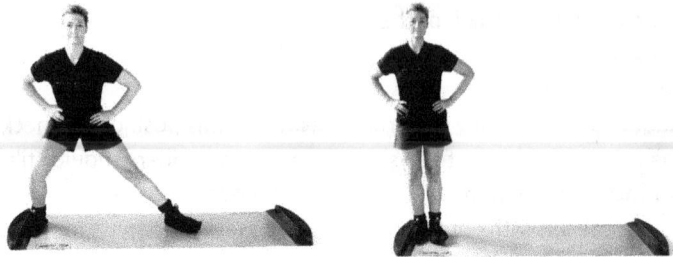

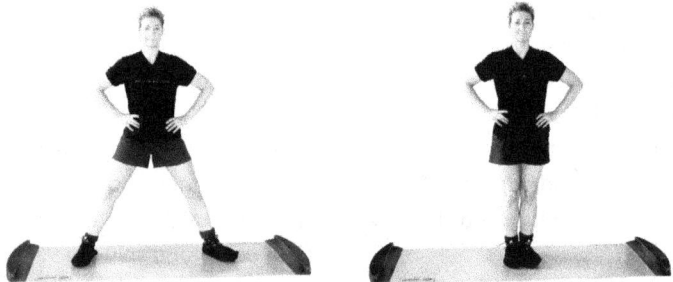

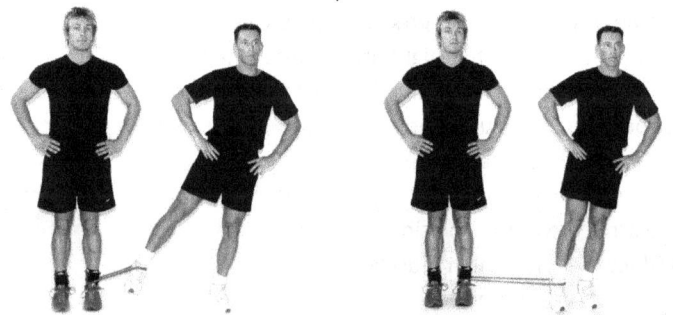

**ADDUCTION
STANDING ON SLIDE**

Primary muscles:
Adductors

**ADDUCTION
STANDING
WITH RUBBERBAND**

Primary muscles:
Adductors

**ADDUCTION, CROSSOVER,
LEG LATERALLY ROTATED,
STANDING WITH
RUBBERBAND**

Primary muscles:
Adductors (pectineus focus)

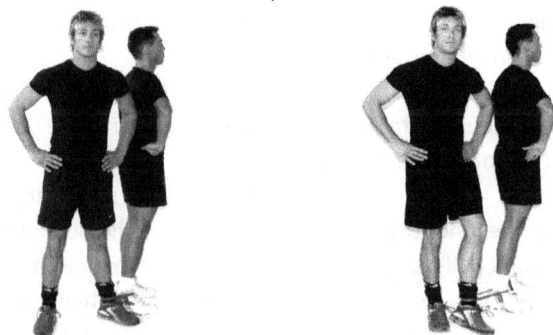

Standing on a slideboard. Slidesocks over the shoes. One foot firmly on the end ramp. The other foot on the slide. Contract the adductors and pull the slide leg in towards the stationary leg.	Slide training and slide exercises are recommended in basic training for skiing. Keep knees aligned with feet. Create resistance by pressing the slide leg towards the slide board.	On the floor with a piece of carpet or cloth under the slide leg.
Standing on the middle of a slideboard. Slidesocks over the shoes. Feet are together. Let the legs slide a little away from each other. Contract the adductors and pull the legs towards each other again. Keep an even pressure on both feet.	Slide training and slide exercises are recommended in basic training for skiing. Keep knees aligned with feet. Create resistance by pressing slide leg into the slide board. Be careful that the legs do not slide too far away from each other.	On the floor with a piece of carpet or cloth under the slide leg.
Standing. Feet are hip-width apart. Rubberband around the ankle and anchored on wall bar or partner. The leg is adducted straight into the opposite, stationary, leg, in the frontal plane. Return with control.	Contract the core muscles to stabilize the body. Keep the lower back and pelvis stable and in neutral, place, so the movement is at the hip.	Different arm and body position. Exercise can be performed without a partner with rubber-band attached to wall bar.
Standing. Rubberband around the ankle and anchored on a wall bar or by partner. Working leg starts from 20 degrees behind the body and In outward rotation. Leg is adducted 20 degr. past the midline of the body and 20 degr. forward, while rotated. Return with control.	Contract the core muscles to stabilize the body. Keep the lower back and pelvis stable and in neutral, so the movement is at the hip.	Different arm and body position. Exercise can be performed without a partner with the rubberband attached to a wall bar.

**ADDUCTION
WITH INTERNAL ROTATION
STANDING WITH
RUBBERBAND**

Primary muscles:
Adductors
(gracilis focus)

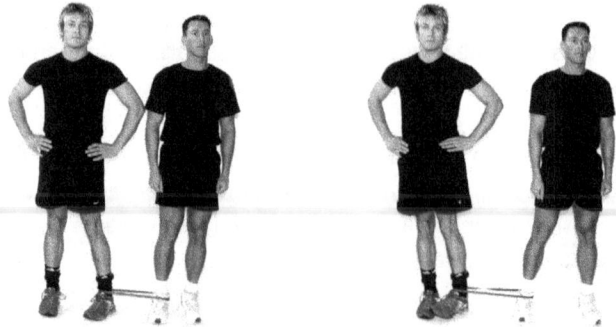

**ADDUCTION, CROSSOVER,
WITH INTERNAL ROTATION,
STANDING WITH
RUBBERBAND**

Primary muscles:
Adductors (adductor longus
and brevis focus)

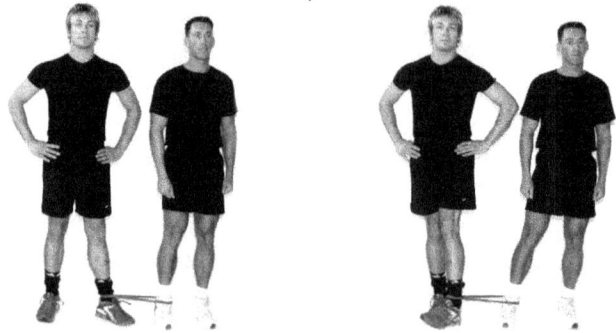

**ADDUCTION
WITH EXTERNAL ROTATION
STANDING WITH
RUBBERBAND**

Primary muscles:
Adductors (adductor magnus,
front fibres focus)

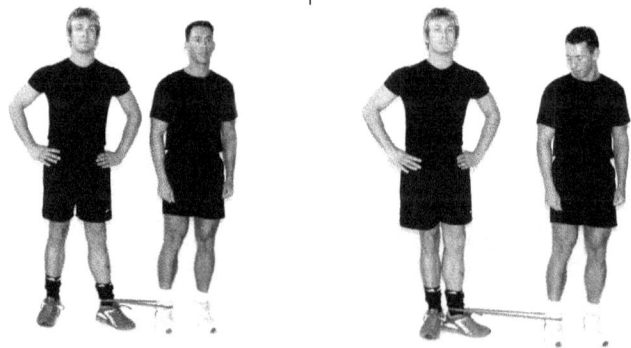

**ABDUCTION
ONE-LEG (UNILATERAL)
STANDING**

Primary muscles:
Gluteus medius and minimus

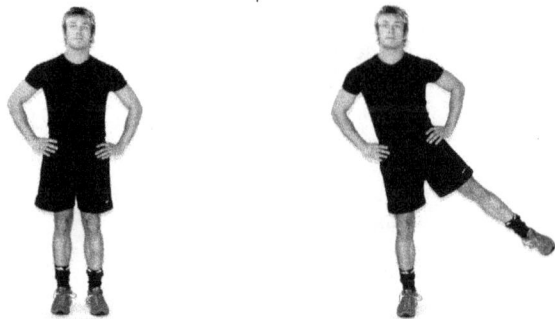

TECHNIQUE	NOTE	VARIATION
Standing. Rubberband around the ankle. Working leg starts in 20 degree abduction. Adduct the leg towards the stationary leg and at the same time rotate the leg inward. Return with control.	Contract the core muscles to stabilize the body. Keep the lower back and pelvis stable and in place, so the movement is at the hip.	Different arm position. Exercise can be performed without a partner with a rubberband attached to a wall bar.
Standing. Rubberband around the ankle. Working leg starts 20 degrees in front of the body and in outward rotation. Adduct the leg front of the opposite leg and at the same time rotate the leg inward. Return with control.	Contract the core muscles to stabilize the body. Keep the lower back and pelvis stable and in place, so the movement is at the hip.	Different arm position. Exercise can be performed without a partner with a rubberband attached to a wall bar.
Standing. Rubberband around the ankle. Working leg is abducted 20 degrees. Adduct the leg to the stationary leg and at the same time rotate the leg outward. Return with control.	Contract the core muscles to stabilize the body. Keep the lower back and pelvis stable and in place, so the movement is at the hip.	Focus adduktor magnus, back fibres: Leg starts 20 degrees in front of the body (hip flexion). Pull the leg backward into hip extension with inward rotation. Exercise can be performed without a partner with a band attached to a wall bar.
Standing on one leg. Working leg is abducted approx. 50 degrees to the side, in the frontal plane. Feet are parallel throughout the exercise. Abduct the working leg without hip rotation. Return to the starting position. Repeat without resting.	Balance work. Contract the core muscles to stabilize the body. Works the abductors at both sides – isometric work for the stationary leg, dynamic work for the working leg.	With or without hiprotation. With or without resistance. **SEVEN** Abduct the leg, hold, do seven pulses, three pure abduction, then four with alternating in- and outward rotation. Lower. Repeat with other leg.

EXERCISE	TECHNIQUE

**SIDESTEP (STEP TOUCH)
WITH RUBBERBAND**

Primary muscles:
Gluteus medius and minimus,
transversus abdominis

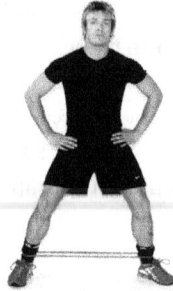

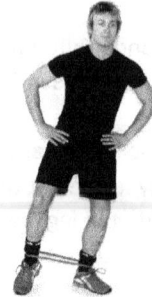

**ABDUCTION/SQUAT
WITH TUBE**

Primary muscles:
Gluteus medius and
minimus

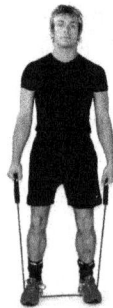

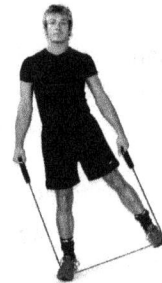

**ABDUCTION/SIDELIFT
WITH TUBE**

Primary muscles:
Gluteus medius and
minimus,
medial deltoid

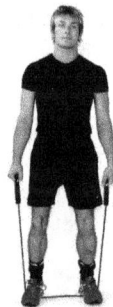

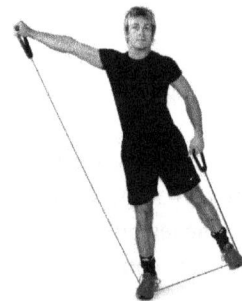

**ABDUCTION/SIDELIFT
WITH RESISTANCE BAND**

Primary muscles:
Gluteus medius and
minimus,
medial and anterior deltoid

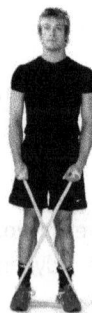

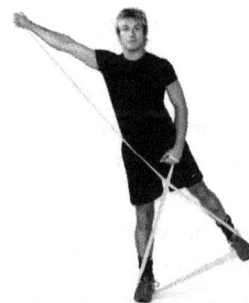

Standing. Rubberband around both ankles. Take a large step to the side. Follow with the other leg, but resist the pull of the rubberband. No slack, ie. legs are not adducted completely. Repeat with opposite leg and return to starting position.	Balance work. Contract the core muscles to stabilize the body.	Different arm movements. Rubberband above or below the knees. In case of knee problems put rubberband above the knees. **DOUBLE STEP TOUCH** Take two steps to the side and two steps back.
Standing. Tube under feet, a tubehandle in each hand. Abduct one leg to the side, return and squat with both legs. Extend the legs and abduct the opposite leg. Repeat.	Balance work. Contract the core muscles to stabilize the body. Works the abductors of both sides – isometric work for the stationary leg, dynamic work for the working leg.	With or without rubberband, tube or band. Different binding.
Standing. Tube under feet, a tubehandle in each hand. Abduct one leg to the side and at the same time the opposite arm performs a lateral raise. Lower. Repeat with opposite leg and shoulder and arm.	Balance work. Contract the core muscles to stabilize the body. Works the abductors of both sides – isometric work for the stationary leg, dynamic work for the working leg.	Different arm movements. With tube or band.
Standing. Resistance band under feet. Band crossed in front of the body. Hold the ends of the band in both hands. Abduct one leg and lift the opposite arm into a high lateral raise. Lower. Repeat with the opposite leg and arm.	Balance work. Contract the core muscles to stabilize the body. Works the abductors of both sides – isometric work for the stationary leg, dynamic work for the working leg.	Different arm movements.

EXERCISE	TECHNIQUE

**ABDUCTION WITH TORSO
ROTATION, STANDING,
UNILATERAL WITH BAND**

Primary muscles:
Gluteus medius and minimus,
transversus abdominis,
obliques internus and externus

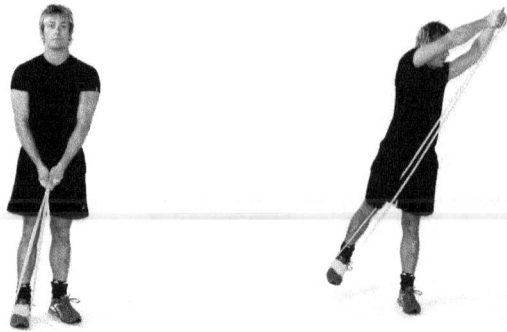

**ABDUCTION, UNILATERAL,
SITTING, ONE LEG
WITH RUBBERBAND**

Primary muscles:
Gluteus medius and minimus,
tensor fascia latae

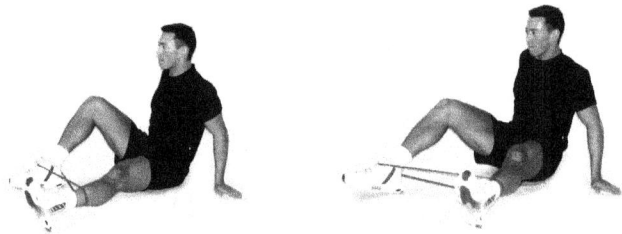

**ABDUCTION
SUPINE
WITH RUBBERBAND**

Primary muscles:
Gluteus medius and minimus

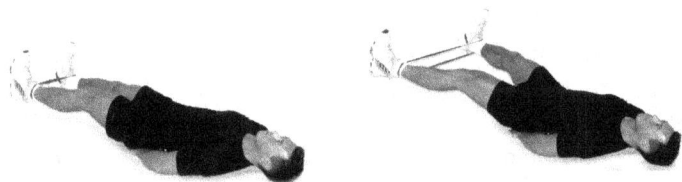

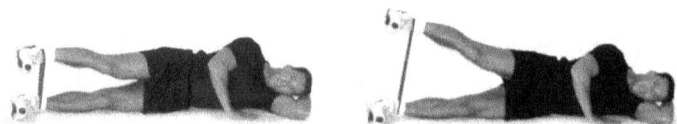

**ABDUCTION
SIDELYING
HIPS AND LEGS STRAIGHT**

Primary muscles:
Gluteus medius and minimus

Standing. Band under one foot. The hands in front of the body. Both hands grip the ends of the band. Abduct the leg, at the same time turn the torso and lift the arms with the band in the opposite direction. Return. Repeat. After a set change side.	Balance work. Works the abductors on both sides – isometric work for the stationary leg, dynamic work for the working leg. Contract the core muscles to stabilize the body.	Differentt range of motion.
Sitting. One leg is flexed and on the floor with rubberband under the foot. The other, working, leg, is straight and just above the floor with a rubberband around the ankle. Abduct the leg. Return. Do not adduct the leg completely, keep the rubberband tension.	Contract the core muscles to stabilize the body. Put both hands on the floor or put hands around the bent leg to stabilize the body.	With or without rotation. With partner resistance.
Supine. Legs are straight and lifted just above the floor, with a rubberband around the ankles. Abduct the legs. Return. Do not adduct the legs completely; keep the rubber band tension.	You can put the hands under the buttocks to tilt the pelvis to keep the lower back comfortably on the floor. In case of knee problems put the rubberband around the thighs right above the knees.	Unilateral, bilateral. With or without rotation. With partner resistance.
Sidelying. Hips are straight, legs are aligned with torso and straight. The head rests on the arm. The other hand is on the floor to stabilize the body. Abduct, lift, the top leg approx. 50 degrees. Lower with control; keep the rubberband tension.	Torso is on the floor with the head on the arm. Or torso is slightly lifted and supported by the forearm. Hips and spine in neutral. In case of knee problems put the rubberband around the thighs right above the knees.	The working leg straight or flexed at the knee (short or long lever). With or without rotation. With or without resistance.

EXERCISE	TECHNIQUE

ABDUCTION
SIDELYING, HIPS AND KNEES
FLEXED 45°

Primary muscles:
Gluteus medius and minimus,
tensor fascia latae

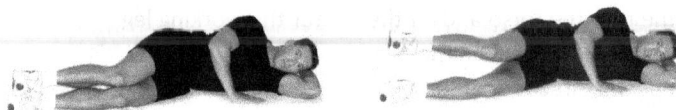

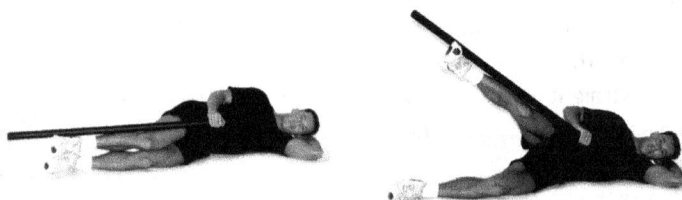

ABDUCTION
SIDELYING
WITH BODYBAR LIFTED

Primary muscles:
Gluteus medius and minimus,
tensor fascia latae

ABDUCTION
SIDELYING
WITH BODYBAR SUPPORTED

Primary muscles:
Gluteus medius and minimus

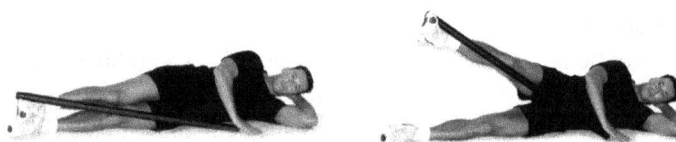

ABDUCTION, HIPS FLEXED,
KNEES STRAIGHT,
SUPINE

Primary muscles:
Gluteus maximus, medius and
minimus, piriformis

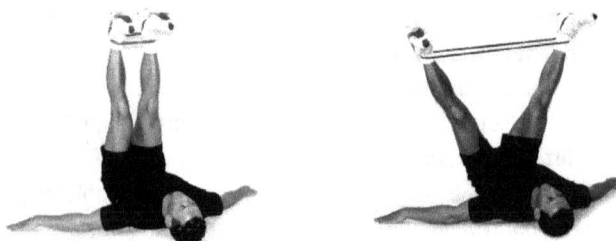

TECHNIQUE	NOTE	VARIATION
Sidelying. Legs are slightly bent at the hip and the knees, approx. 45 degrees. The hands are on the floor to stabilize the body. Abduct the top leg approx. 50 degrees. Lower with control.	Torso is on the floor with the head on the arm. Or torso is slightly lifted and supported by the forearm. Note: In this position the neck and the shoulders should still be in neutral position. Keep hips and spine in neutral position.	The working leg is straight or bent. With or without rotation: The leg can be rotated inward and outward during the exercise. With or without rubberband or dumbbell. On floor, bench or ball.
Sidelying. Legs are slightly bent at the hip and the knees. A bodybar rests on the top leg, on three points: Foot, lower leg, thigh. Hold bar in place with the top hand. Abduct the leg. Lower leg with control, do not let it rest on the bottom leg.	Torso is on the floor with the head on the arm. Or torso is slightly lifted and supported by the forearm. Note: In this position the neck and the shoulders should still be in neutral position. Keep hips and spine in neutral position.	Different leg position, top leg.
Sidelying. Legs are straight. A bodybar rests on the top foot. The other end is on the floor (if needed keep the bodybar steady with the hand). Abduct the leg. Lower leg with control, do not let it rest on the bottom leg.	Rest torso on the floor with the head on the arm or the floor. Or lift the torso and rest on the forearm. Note: In this position the neck and the shoulders should still be in neutral position. Keep hips and spine in neutral position.	Different leg position, top leg.
Supine. Leg straight and vertical. Rubberband around the ankles. Legs are abducted to the side, away from each other. Return with control. Avoid adducting the legs completely, keep the rubber band tension.	You can put the hands under the buttocks to tilt the pelvis to keep the lower back comfortably on the floor.	With rubberband over or under the knee. With partner resistance. The legs at different angles to the body.

EXERCISE	TECHNIQUE

**THREE-LEGGED
CALF RAISE**

Primary muscles:
Gastrocnemeus and soleus

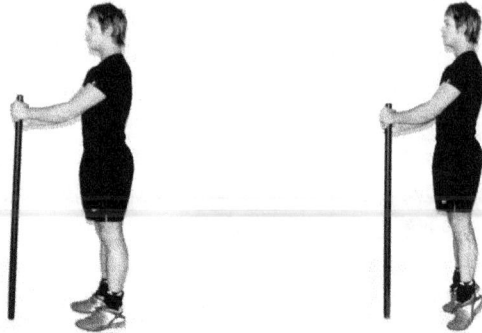

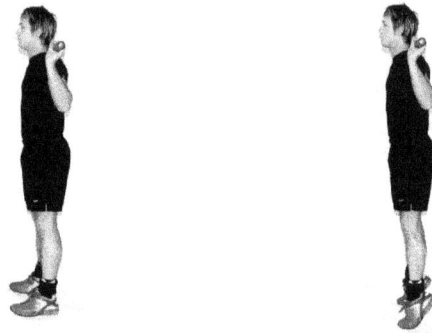

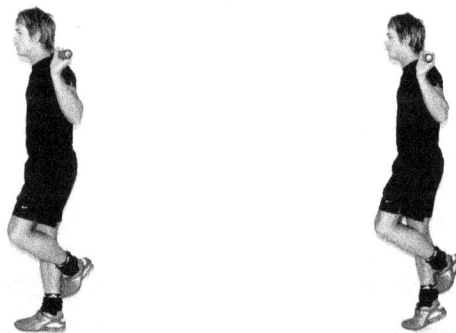

**CALF RAISE
STRAIGHT LEGS**

Primary muscles:
Gastrocnemeus and soleus

ONE-LEG CALF RAISE

Primary muscles:
Gastrocnemeus and soleus

**CALF RAISE
BENT LEGS**

Primary muscles:
Gastrocnemeus and soleus
(focus on soleus)

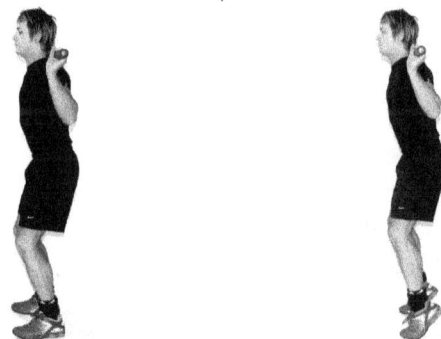

Standing. Feet together or hip-width apart. Hold a barbell/bar in front of the body as a support. Lift the heels and raise the body. Lower with control. Repeat without resting.	Contract the core muscles to stabilize the body.	Different leg position, legs/feet rotated out or in. **DONKEY CALF RAISE** Standing. Torso forward and supported with partner on the back. Straight or bent legs. Calf raise.
Standing. Feet together or hip- or shoulder-width apart. Lift the heels and raise the body. Lower with control. Repeat without resting.	Balance work. Contract the core muscles to stabilize the body.	Different arm positions. Different leg position: Legs rotated out, focus gastrocnemeus medial head. Legs rotated in, focus lateral head. With or without resistance.
Standing. On one leg. Lift the heel and raise the body. Lower with control. Repeat without resting.	Balance work. Contract the core muscles to stabilize the body.	Different arm positions. Different leg position, leg/foot rotated out or in. Different leg position free leg. With or without barbell/dumbbell/ball.
Standing. Feet together or hip- or shoulder-width apart. Legs are slightly bent. Lift the heels and raise the body. Lower with control. Repeat without resting.	Balance work. The center of gravity should move up and down, not just the knees moving forwards and backwards. Contract the core muscles to stabilize the body.	Different arm positions. With or without barbell/dumbbell/ball.

**ONE-LEG CALF RAISE
BENT LEG**

Primary muscles:
Gastrocnemeus and soleus
(focus on soleus)

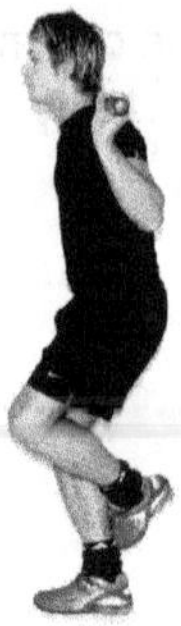

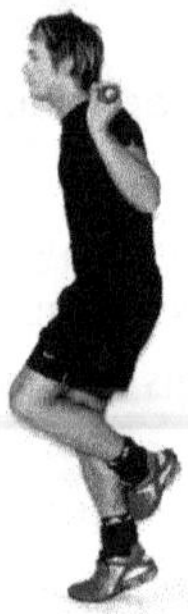

**CALF RAISE
ON THE EDGE OF BENCH**

Primary muscles:
Gastrocnemeus and soleus

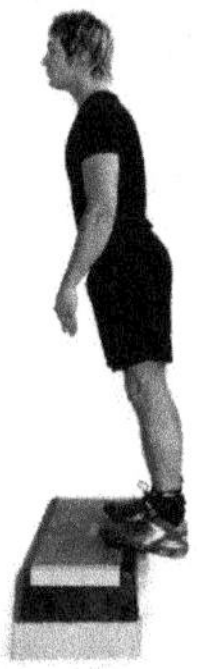

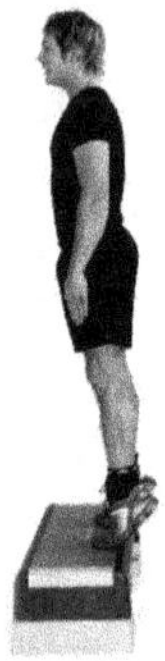

**CALF RAISE, ONE LEG
WITH SUPPORT**

Primary muscles:
Gastrocnemeus and soleus
(focus on soleus)

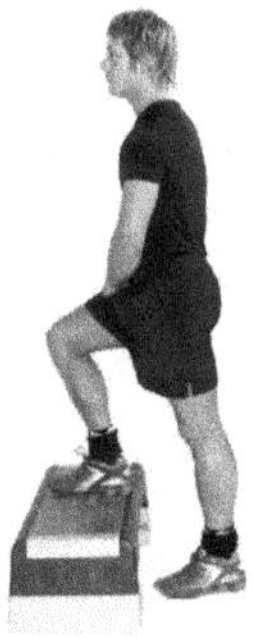

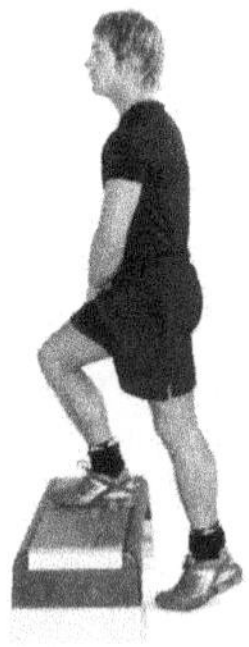

SEATED CALF RAISE

Primary muscles:
Gastrocnemeus and soleus
(focus on soleus)

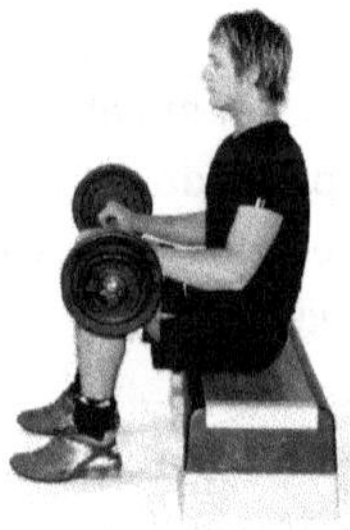

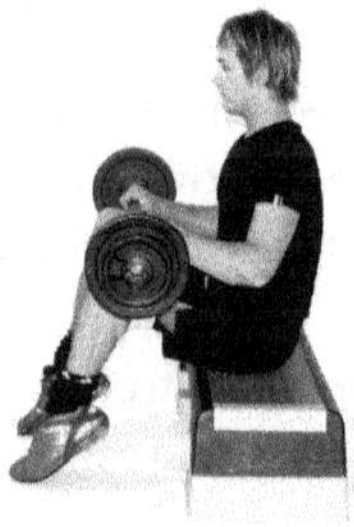

Standing. On one leg. Leg is slightly bent. Lift the heel and raise the body. Lower with control. Repeat without resting.	Balance work. Contract the core muscles to stabilize the body. The center of gravity should move up and down, not just the knees moving forwards and backwards.	Different leg position, free leg. With or without barbell/dumbbell/ball.
Standing. On a bench with heels off the edge. Lower the heels down. Lift the heels and raise the body (up on the toes). Lower with control. Repeat without resting.	The bench must be stable. Avoid lowering the heels too much; do not go beyond normal range of motion, protect the akilles tendon. Balance work.	With or without support (eg. barbell/bar on top of bench). With or without barbell/dumbbell/ball.
Standing. Close behind bench. The working leg is on the floor close to the bench, the other foot supports lightly on the top, do not transfer bodyweight to the top leg. Lift the heel and raise the body. Lower with control. Repeat without resting.	The bodyweight should be centered over the working leg. (not between the legs, as seen on the photo). Balance work.	Different arm exercises. With or without barbell/dumbbell/ball.
Sitting. On bench with bent legs Dumbbell or barbell rest on the thighs. Lift the heels, the legs, against the resistance. Lower with control. Repeat without resting.	Put a towel on the legs, so the barbell does not cut into the thighs.	Different arm exercises. With a barbell or heavy dumbbells.

EXERCISE	TECHNIQUE

**PLANTARFLEXION
SUPINE**

Primary muscles:
Gastrocnemeus and soleus

**DORSILFLEXION,
SUPINE**

Primary muscles:
Tibialis anterior

**DORSIFLEXION
SITTING
WITH RUBBERBAND**

Primary muscles:
Tibialis anterior

**DORSIFLEXION
STANDING TOE RAISE**

Primary muscles:
Tibialis anterior

Supine. Legs vertical. Contract the calf muscles, so the ankle is extended, plantarflexed. Return. Repeat.	Very easy exercise. The exercise helps return the blood from the legs to the torso, eases the pressure on the pelvic floor.	On floor or bench.
Supine. Legs vertical. Contract the shin muscles, so the foot is pulled towards the shins, dorsiflexion. Return. Repeat.	Very easy exercise. The exercise helps return the blood from the legs to the torso, eases the pressure on the pelvic floor.	Different arm position. Different leg position.
Sitting. Rubberband anchored under the stationary leg and over the forefoot of the working leg. Keep the leg lifted to create tension in the rubberband. Bend the ankle, dorsiflexion, so the toes are pulled upwards towards the shin. Lower with control.	The rubberband must be over the toes. If the rubberband is around the ankle, then the band provides no resistance.	Different arm position. Different leg position.
Standing. Lift forefoot, dorsiflexion, so the toes are pulled upwards towards the shin. Lower with control.	Very easy exercise. Can be performed with a bodybar resting on the toes. It is not an optimal variation, however, and it should be avoided, that the bodybar pinches the nerves on top of the foot.	Unilateral, bilateral. With or without resistance. **REVERSE CALF RAISE** Support from bodybar, wall bar or partner. Stand on abench, lower toes down past the edge, pull toes upwards towards the shins. Repeat.

EXERCISE	TECHNIQUE

INVERSION

Primary muscles:
Tibialis anterior,
tibialis posterior

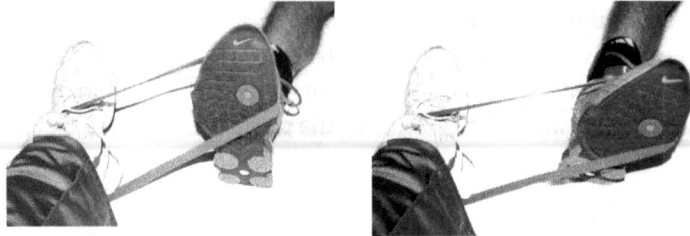

EVERSION

Primary muscles:
Peroneus longus,
peroneus brevis

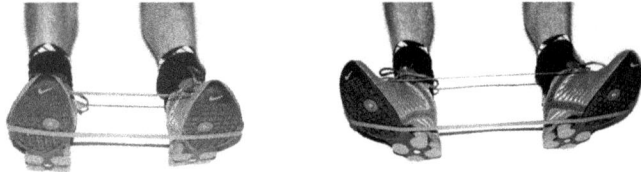

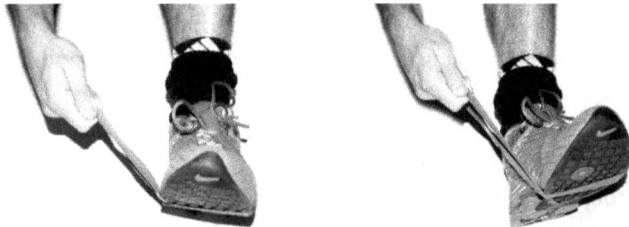

PRONATION

Primary muscles:
Peroneus longus,
peroneus brevis

SUPINATION

Primary muscles:
Tibialis anterior andposterior,
flexor digitorum longus,
flexor hallucis longus

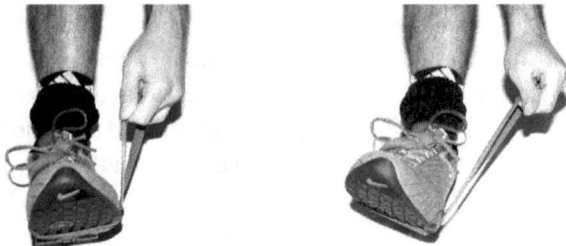

TECHNIQUE	LOGIC	VARIATION
Sitting. On a bench with lower leg resting on bench. Ankle and foot unsupported. Rubbergand around one foot – anchored by a partner or wall bar. The lower leg rotates toward the midline of the body. Return with control.	Exercises for the feet and lower legs are important, as they support the entire body.	Walk on differentt surfaces with different foot positions.
Sitting. On bench with the lower legs resting on bench. Ankle and foot unsupported. Rubberband around the feet. The lower legs rotate outward Away from the midline of the body. Return with control.	Exercises for the feet and lower legs are important, as they support the entire body.	Walk on differentt surfaces with different foot positions.
Sitting. The rubberband is anchored in the shoelaces and under the foot from the outside and up on the inside of the foot. The foot pushes down on the resistance with the inside of the foot. Return with control.	Exercises for the feet and lower legs are important, as they support the entire body.	Walk on differentt surfaces with different foot positions.
Sitting. The rubberband is anchored in the shoelaces and under the foot from the inside and up on the outside of the foot. The foot pushes down on the resistance with the outside of the foot. Return with control.	Exercises for the feet and lower legs are important, as they support the entire body.	Walk on differentt surfaces with different foot positions.

WALKING VARIATIONS

Primary muscles:
Foot and lower leg
muscles

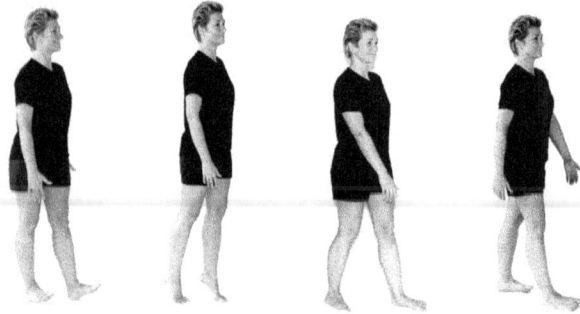

TOE FLEXION

Primary muscles:
Toe flexors,
foot and lower leg
muscles

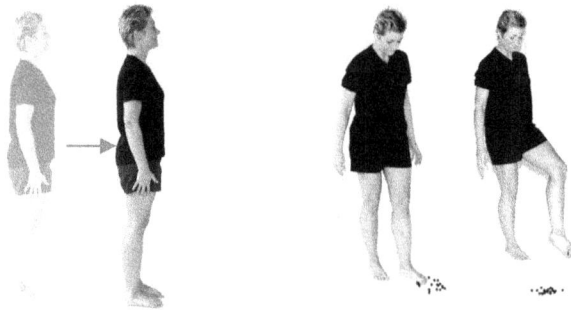

TOE EXTENSION

Primary muscles:
Toe extensors,
foot and lower leg
muscles

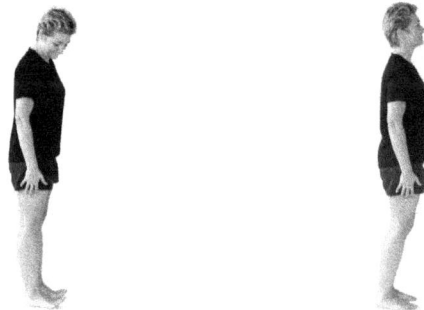

**BALANCING ON
BOARD**

Primary muscles:
Foot and lower legs
muscles,
core muscles

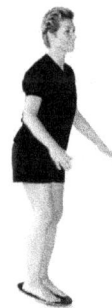

TECHNIQUE		
Walk with the feet in different angles and positions. On the heels, on the toes, on the inside and the outside of the foot.	The exercise can be performed with bare feet or with shoes.	Different surfaces.
Standing. Bend the toes, pull on the carpet to pull the body forward. Release. Repeat. Standing. Bare feet. Bend the toes and pick up marbles from the floor. Pick them up and put them down somewhere else. Repeat.	The exercise should be done on a wall-to-wall carpet. Perform the exercise with bare feet.	Different surfaces. Different objects are collected.
Standing. Pull toes upwards and outwards as high as possible. Extension. Relax and repeat.	Perform the exercise with bare feet.	Different surfaces. Standing or sitting.
Standing on a teeter board. Rock forward and backward. Make circular movements. Keep balance on both legs. Keep balance on one leg.	The exercises can be performed with bare feet or with shoes on. There are different types of teeter boards with various levels of difficulty. Air discs, therapy boards and balls are also recommended.	Different teeter boards and balance equipment. Feet wide apart, together or on one leg. With eyes open or closed.

8 | Lower Back Exercises

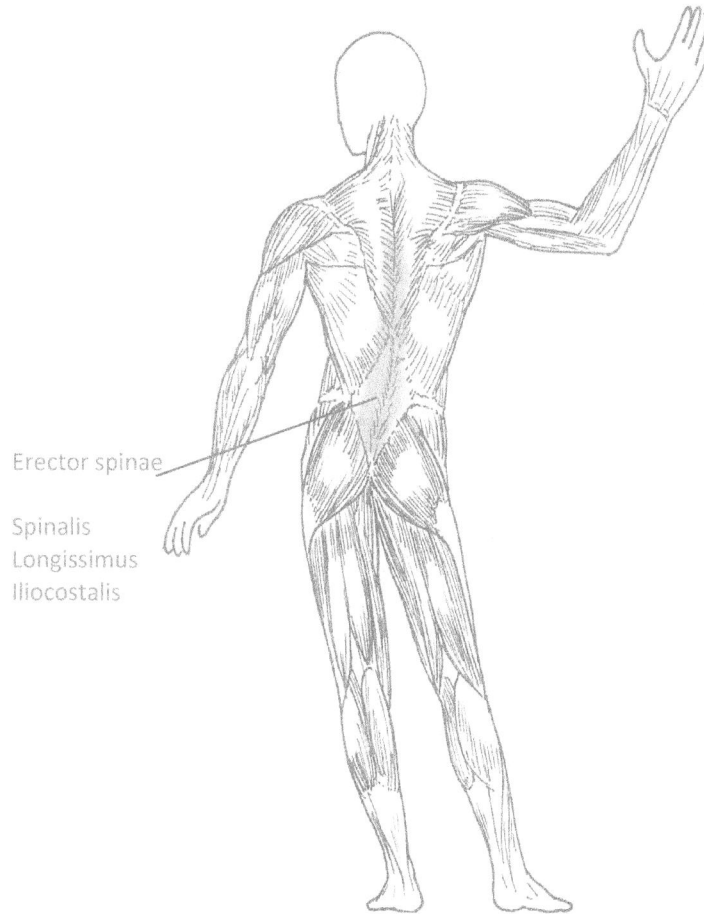

Erector spinae

Spinalis
Longissimus
Iliocostalis

EXERCISE	TECHNIQUE	

**BACK EXTENSION
ARMS DOWN BY THE SIDE**

Primary muscles:
Erector spinae

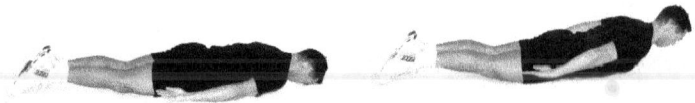

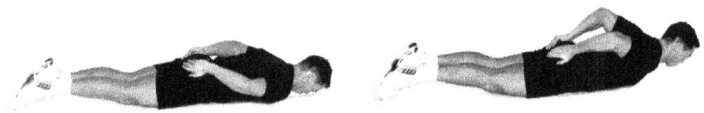

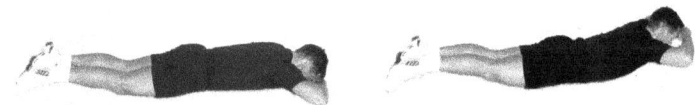

**BACK EXTENSION,
HANDS ON LOWER
BACK/BUTTOCKS**

Primary muscles:
Erector spinae

**BACK EXTENSION,
HANDS BY THE HEAD**

Primary muscles:
Erector spinae

**BACK EXTENSION WITH
TORSO MOVEMENT**

Primary muscles:
Erector spinae

Prone. The neck is in neutral position. Legs together, buttocks and thighs are contracted. The arms at sides on the floor. Contract the back extensors, lift the upper body with control. Lower with control.	The back hyperextends slightly, but without extreme movement. No pain must be experienced. The neck should be in neutral position, not backwards. Contract transversus abdominis to stabilze.	Different leg position. On floor, bench or ball. Breathing pattern: Inhale when lifting, exhale when lowering. Or: Inhale when prone, exhale when lifting, inhale in top position, exhale when lowering.
Prone. The neck is in neutral position. Legs together, buttocks and thighs are contracted. The hands are on the buttocks, elbows are to the side. Contract the back extensors, lift the upper body with control and pull the elbows together. Lower with control.	The back hyper-extends slightly, but without extreme movement. No pain must be experienced. The neck should be in neutral, not backwards. Contract the transversus abdominis to stabilize.	Different arm position. In top position the shoulder blades can be adducted, pull the elbows towards each other. Different leg position.
Prone. The neck is in neutral position. Legs together, buttocks and thighs are contracted. The arms at sides on the floor. Contract the back extensors, lift the upper body with control. Lower with control.	The back extends, that is it hyper-extends slightly, but without extreme movement. No pain must be experienced. The neck should be in neutral, not backwards. Contract the transversus abdominis to stabilze.	Different arm/body/leg position. With or without resistance: Dumbbells by the shoulders. With a barbell on top of the back. Note: Not on the neck.
Prone. Legs together, buttocks and thighs are contracted. Neck in neutral position. Arms are forward on the floor on each side of the head. Contract the back extensors, lift the upper body with control. Lift the arms in up, out and back. Lower with control.	The back extends, that is it hyper-extends slightly, but without extreme movement. No pain must be experienced. The neck should be in neutral, not backwards. Contract the transversus abdominis to stabilze.	Different arm movements. Different leg position. With or without resistance.

179

EXERCISE	TECHNIQUE

**BACK EXTENSION
ARMS OVERHEAD**

Primary muscles:
Erector spinae

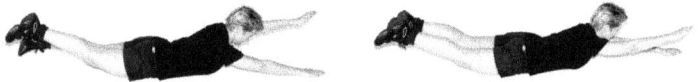

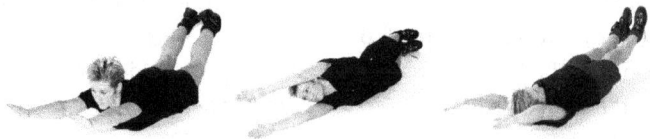

**BACK EXTENSION,
ISOMETRIC,
WITH ARM-LEG-LIFT
(SWIMMING, FLUTTER)**

Primary muscles:
Erector spinae

**BACK EXTENSION
SIDE ROLL TO
ABDOMINAL CURL**

Primary muscles:
Erector spinae

**BACK EXTENSION
WITH ROTATION
PRONE**

Primary muscles:
Erector spinae, rotators,
multifidii

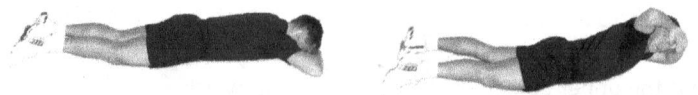

Prone. The neck is in neutral position. Legs are together. The arms straight forward – hands on top of each other; upper arms support the head. Lift the torso, extend with control. Lower with control.	The back extends, that is it hyper-extends slightly, but without extreme movement. No pain must be experienced. The neck should be in neutral, not backwards. Buttocks and thighs may be contracted to stabilize pelvis.	One or both arms forward. Different leg position. With or without resistance. **SUPERMAN** Prone. Core muscles contract. Lift the legs and the arms with control. Lower.
Prone. The neck is in neutral position. Legs are together and lifted. Arms are forward and lifted. The torso is liftet into back extension. Hold. Arms and legs move up and down with small, fast flutter movements.	The back extends, that is it hyper-extends slightly, but without extreme movement. No pain must be experienced. The neck should be in neutral, not backwards.	One or both arms forward. Different leg position. With or without resistance.
Prone. Legs together. Thigh muscles are contracted, so the knees are liftet off the floor. Arms are forward. Contract the back extensors, lift the upper body, back extension. Lower. Roll sideways ½ or 1½ turn into supine position. Ab curl. Lower. Roll back. Repeat.	Combination exercise, a nice variation or transition. The back extends, that is it hyper-extends slightly, but without extreme movement. No pain must be experienced. The neck should be in neutral, not backwards.	One or both arms forward. Different leg position. With or without resistance.
Prone. The neck is in neutral position. Feet on the floor. Legs are together. Arms at sides or hands under the forehead. Lift the upper body, rotate to the side, back to center, lower with control. Repeat with rotation to the opposite side.	The back extends, that is it hyper-extends slightly, but without extreme movement. No pain must be experienced. The neck should be in neutral, not backwards. Four phases: Up, rotate to the side, rotate back, down.	Different leg position. On floor, bench or ball.

EXERCISE	TECHNIQUE

**BACK EXTENSION
WITH SIDEBEND
PRONE**

Primary muscles:
Erector spinae, obliques

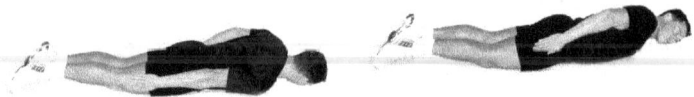

**DIAGONAL LIFT
PRONE**

Primary muscles:
Erector spinae, multifidii,
rotators

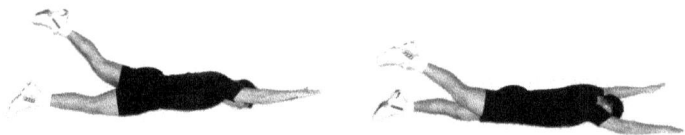

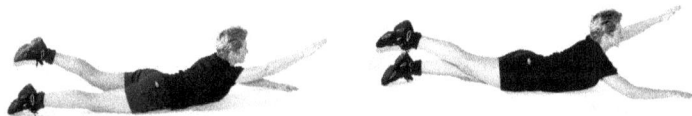

**BACK EXTENSION WITH
DIAGONAL LIFT**

Primary muscles:
Erector spinae, multifidii,
rotators

**DIAGONAL LIFT
(QUADRUPED)
ON ALL FOURS**

Primary muscles:
Erector spinae, multifidii,
transversus abdominis,
rotators

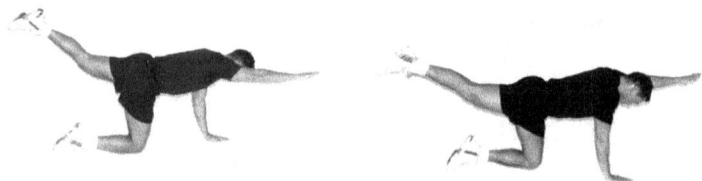

Prone. Neck in neutral. Legs together, buttocks and thighs contracted. Arms on the floor along the side of the body. Contract the back extensors, lift the upper body with control. In this position bend to the side and return. Lower with control.	The back hyper-extends slightly, but without extreme movement. No pain must be experienced. The neck should be in neutral, not backwards. Four phases: Up, sidebend, return, down. In frontal plane.	Different leg position. On floor, bench or ball.
Prone. The forehead on the floor. The arms are forward by the sides of the head. Lift one arm and the opposite leg. Lower with control. Repeat with the opposite arm and leg.	The exercise is a diagonal lift exercise, which activates the multifidii and rotators. It is an entry level strength and stability exercise as you are supported on the floor; for beginners or people with poor balance.	On floor, bench or ball. The torso can be lifted at the same time. Alternate or repeat with the same arm and leg.
Prone. The arms are forward. Lift the upper body into back extension. Lift one arm and the opposite leg. Lower with control Repeat with the opposite arm and leg.	The exercise is a diagonal lift exercise, which activates the multifidii and rotators. Avoid uncontrolled, ballistic, movement of the arms and legs to protect the back.	On floor, bench or ball. Alternate or repeat with the same arm and leg.
On all fours. (Six points of support: Hands, knees and feet). The neck is in neutral position. The core muscles contract. One arm and the opposite leg lift to or just past horizontal. Lower with control. Repeat with opposite arm and leg.	Excellent core- and balance exercise. The neck should be in neutral, not backwards. Alternate or repeat with the same arm and leg.	On floor, bench or ball. **TWO-POINT DIAGONAL LIFT** Increase the difficulty by lifting the lower leg from the floor, so the base of support is smaller. **SAME SIDE ARM-LEG LIFT** Lift same side arm and leg. Try to keep the hips level.

EXERCISE	TECHNIQUE

**DIAGONAL LIFT
ON ALL FOURS
ELBOW TO KNEE**

Primary muscles:
Gluteus maximus, hamstrings,
erector spinae, rotators,
transversus abd., multifidii

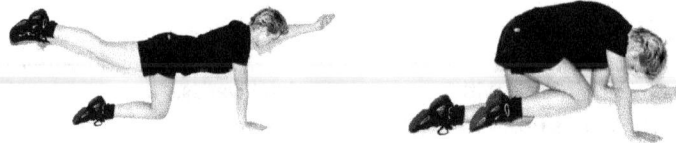

**DIAGONAL LIFT
ON ALL FOURS
ARM/LEG ABDUCTION**

Primary muscles:
Erector spinae, hamstrings,
gluteus maximus, rotators,
transversus abd., multifidii

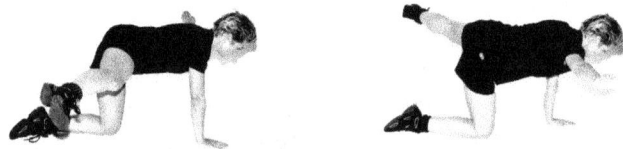

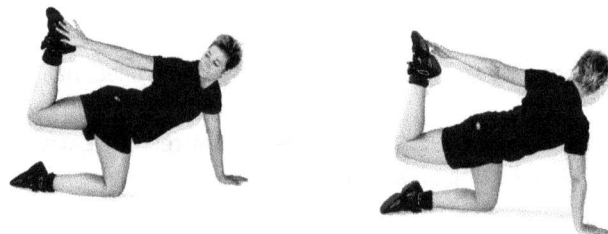

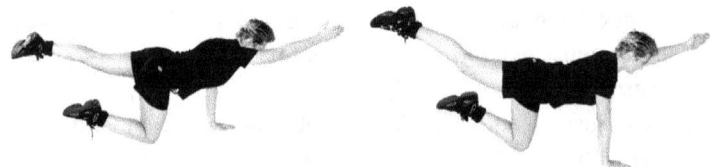

**DIAGONAL LIFT
ON ALL FOURS
HAND TO FOOT**

Primary muscles:
Erector spinae, hamstrings,
gluteus maximus, rotators,
transversus abd., multifidii

**DIAGONAL LIFT
ON ALL FOURS
KNEE SUPPORT**

Primary muscles:
Erector spinae, hamstrings,
gluteus maximus, rotators,
transversus abd., multifidii

TECHNIQUE	FOCUS	VARIATION
On all fours. Opposite arm and leg lift to horizontal or slightly above. Pull elbow and knee toward each other. Return. Arm and leg are lowered. Repeat with the opposite side.	Contract the core muscles to stabilize the body. Neck in neutral position. Turn the thumb towards the ceiling, when the arm lifts, to avoid shoulder impingement.	On floor or ball. Different leg position. With or without resistance.
On all fours. Opposite arm and leg lift to horizontal or slightly above. In horizontal plane move the arm and the leg sideways, in horizontal plane, away from the midline of the body. Move arm and leg back in. Lower arm and leg. Repeat with the opposite side.	Contract the core muscles to stabilize the body. Neck in neutral position. Turn the thumb towards the ceiling, when the arm lifts, to avoid shoulder impingement.	On floor or ball. Different leg position. With or without resistance.
On all fours. Opposite arm and leg lift. Bend the leg and the arm, touch the hand to the foot. Extend arm and leg back out. Lower arm and leg. Repeat with the opposite side.	Contract the core muscles to stabilize the body. Neck in neutral position. Turn the thumb towards the ceiling, when the arm lifts, to avoid shoulder impingement.	On floor or ball. With or without resistance.
On all fours. Opposite arm and leg lift. Lift the lower leg of the supporting leg for increased difficulty, area of support is smaller. Hold for a second. Lower arm and leg. Repeat with the opposite side.	You can put a towel under the knee, it is more comfortable. Contract the core muscles. Neck in neutral position. Turn the thumb towards the ceiling, when the arm lifts, to avoid shoulder impingement.	On floor or ball. With or without resistance.

EXERCISE	TECHNIQUE

**DIAGONAL LIFT,
PLANK POSITION
ELBOW TO KNEE**

Primary muscles:
Gluteus maximus, hamstrings,
erector spinae, rotators,
transversus abd., multifidii

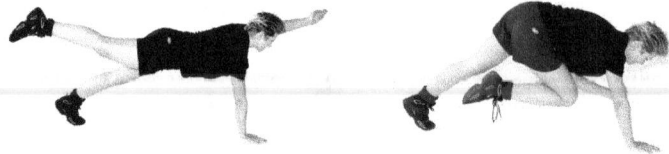

**BACK EXTENSION
WITH ARM CHANGE
PRONE**

Primary muscles:
Erector spinae, hamstrings,
gluteus maximus

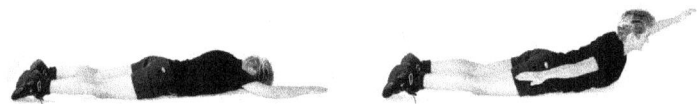

**BACK EXTENSION
DIAGONAL LIFT
WITH SIDE BEND
PRONE**

Primary muscles:
Erector spinae, hamstrings,
gluteus maximus, obliques

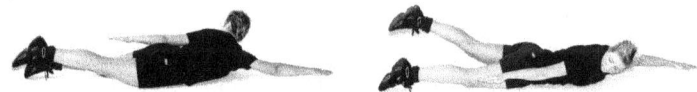

PARACHUTE (FLYER)

Primary muscles:
Erector spinae

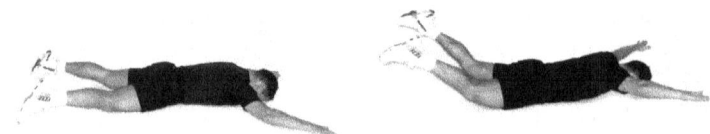

Plank position. On the hands and toes. Opposite arm and leg lift. Pull elbow and knee towards each other. Return. Lower arm and leg. Repeat with opposite arm and leg.	For advanced exercisers. Contract the core muscles to stabilize the body. Neck in neutral position (on photo head is lifted slightly). Turn the thumb towards the ceiling, when the arm lifts, to avoid shoulder impingement.	Different leg position.
Prone. One arm is at the side of the torso, the other forward by the side of the head. Contract the back extensors, lift upper body, while arms change position. Lower. Repeat with the opposite side.	Contract the core muscles to stabilize the body. Neck in neutral position (on photo head is lifted slightly). Turn the thumb towards the ceiling, when the arm lifts, to avoid shoulder impingement.	Different arm position. Different leg position. With or without resistance.
Prone. The arms are forward by the side of the head. The upper body lifts and the opposite arm and leg lift. Sidebend the torso and the lifted arm towards the stationary leg. Return. Repeat with the opposite side.	Contract the core muscles to stabilize the body. Neck in neutral position.	Different arm position. Different leg position.
Prone. The arms are forward, outward and lifted. The legs are slightly bent and abducted, out, and lifted from the floor as in a 'parachute jump'. Hold position isometrically for as long as desired.	Remember to keep breathing. Neck is in neutral position.	Different arm position. Isometric or dynamic exercise.

EXERCISE	TECHNIQUE

HIP EXTENSION

Primary muscles:
Gluteus maximus, hamstrings,
erector spinae

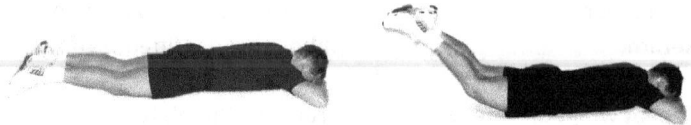

**BACK EXTENSION AND
HIP EXTENSION
(ROCK THE BOAT)**

Primary muscles:
Erector spinae, the hamstrings,
gluteus maximus

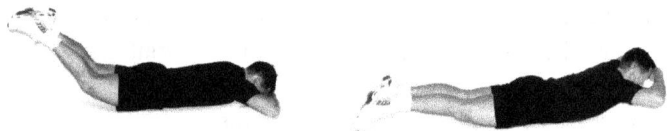

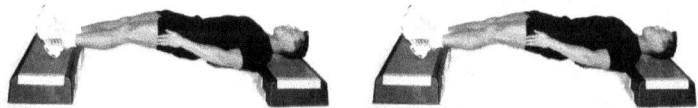

**REVERSE PLANK
BETWEEN TWO BENCHES**

Primary muscles:
Erector spinae, hamstrings,
gluteus maximus

**NECK PRESS
SUPINE**

Primary muscles:
Trapezius (upper part),
sternocleidomastoideus
and other neck muscles

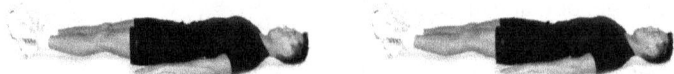

Prone. Forehead on the floor. Hands down by the side or under the head. Leg lift from the floor. (In the top position the buttocks and lower back may contract even harder, so the hips lift from the floor). Legs are lowered with control.	The core muscles contract. Works the buttocks and the hamstrings, as well as the lower back muscles. Lifting hips may be hard on lower back and is not recommended for people with back problems.	On floor, bench or ball. Different leg position. With or without resistance.
Prone. The torso is lifted and lowered. Immediately after the torso is on the floor, the legs are lifted and lowered. This is a smooth continuus movement without pausing.	Lift upper or lower body, not boty at the same time, this is a 'rocking' movement. Preparation, practice technique: 2 torso lifts, 2 leg lifts > 1 torso lift, 1 leg lift > '½ lifts', 'rock the boat' motion.	Different arm position. Arms at sides, by the head or forward, overhead. Different leg position. With or without resistance.
Supine. The upper back is supported on a bench and the feet/heels on another bench. The body forms a 'bridge' between the two benches. The back extensors and buttocks contract to maintain this bridge position.	Supoort is on the upper back muscles. Avoid supporting on the neck.	Different arm position. Different leg position. With one or both legs resting on the bench. On the floor, with heels and upper back resting.
Supine. Legs together. Arms at sides. The body is relaxed – or contract the core muscles – neutral lower back. Hold the tongue to the roof of the mouth. Press the back of the head i nto the floor, create resistance, make a 'long neck' with neck in neutral. Relax.	The body is relaxed – or contract the core muscles – neutral lower back. Hold the position isometrically for 5-30 seconds (or longer).	Focus on posture and muscle control.

EXERCISE	TECHNIQUE

**BACK ROLL UP
KNEELING**

Primary muscles:
Erector spinae

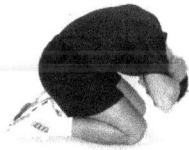

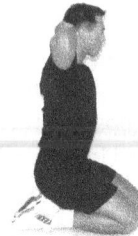

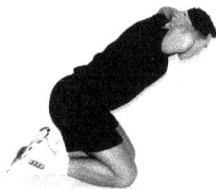

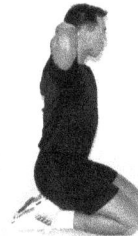

**BACK EXTENSION
KNEELING**

Primary muscles:
Erector spinae

**CAT-CAMEL EXERCISE
ON ALL FOURS**

Primary muscles:
Erector spinae,
rectus abdominis

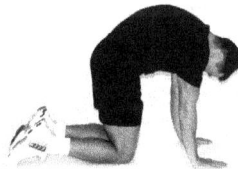

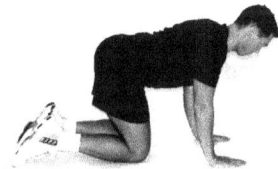

**TORSO ROTATION
ON ALL FOURS**

Primary muscles:
Rotators, multifidii,
transversus abdominis

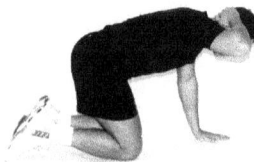

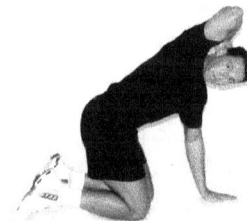

Kneeling. The arms at sides or behind the head. Lower the torso forward over the legs. Keep contracting, do not relax or pause. Contract the back extensors and raise the torso, extend the spine, one vertebrae at a time.	Contract the core muscles to stabilize the body. Good exercise, but may be uncomfortable for the knees.	Different arm position. Bend over with a straight back body or roll down.
Kneeling. The arms at sides or behind the head. Lower the torso forward over the legs. Keep contracting, do not relax or pause. Contract the back extensors and raise the torso, extend the spine – as one unit.	Contract the core muscles to stabilize the body. Good exercise, but may be uncomfortable for the knees.	Different arm position.
On all fours. Forearms or hands on the floor. Lower legs on the floor. Contract the abdominals and arch the back. Release with control. Smooth continuus movement without pauses.	An excellent exercise form mobility, posture and breathing. Coordinate with your breathing; inhale and arch the back, exhale and sag the back.	Different arm position. The hands/forearms on a bench, various heights. Pause, with contraction, in the end ranges of motion.
On all fours. One forearm or hand on the floor. The other hand supported on the head. Rotate the torso to the side of the arm behind the head. Spine, neck and head rotate together; you look to the side. Lower with control back to neutral position. Repeat.	For strength and flexibility. An excellent back exercise, which brings attention to the torso and core muscles. After a set, change side.	Different arm position. You can hold a dumbbell at the elbow joint, held by the upper arm and forearm, providing slightly increased resistance.

EXERCISE	TECHNIQUE

**CAT-CAMEL EXERCISE
STANDING, SUPPORTED**

Primary muscles:
Erector spinae,
transversus abdominis

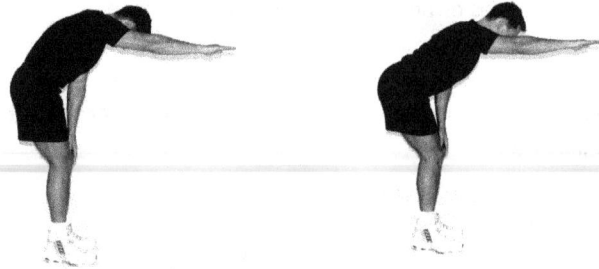

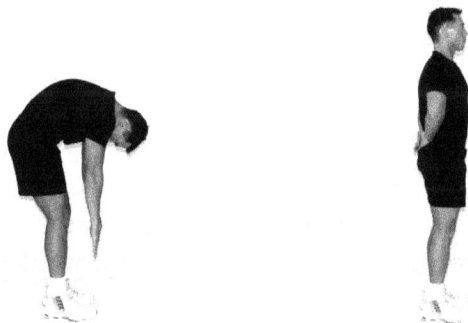

**CAT-CAMEL EXERCISE
STANDING, UNSUPPORTED**

Primary muscles:
Erector spinae,
transversus abdominis,
rectus abdominis

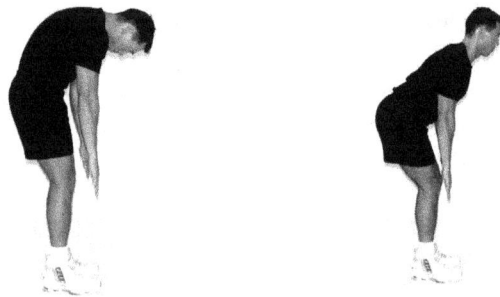

**BACK ROLL UP
STANDING**

Primary muscles:
Erector spinae,
transversus abdominis

BACK EXTENSION STANDING

Primary muscles:
Erector spinae,
gluteus maximus, hamstrings,
transversus abdominis

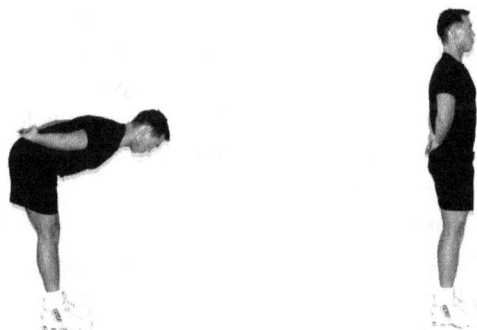

TECHNIQUE	NOTE	VARIATION
Standing. Legs together or hip-width apart. Hands support on the thigh. Raise one arm to horizontal. Lower and change arm. Contract the core muscles to stabilize. Do a cat-camel movement. Arch and release.	Contract the core muscles to stabilize the body. Instead of doing the cat-camel movement, just keep the position for as long as desired. After a set, change the arm.	Different arm/leg position. Focus on either the transversus abdominis, flatten your abs, or on the back extensors. Or both.
Standing. Legs together or hip-width apart. The hands in front of the body without supporting on the legs. Abdominal and back muscles (back extensors) contract alternatingly to bend and extend the lower back.	Contract the core muscles to stabilize the body. The erector spinae, back extensors, are the prime movers. The rectus abdominis is not working against gravity.	Different arm/leg position.
Standing. Legs together or hip-width apart. Legs slightly bent. Upper body is curled forward. Hands in front of the legs. Contract the back extensors and raise the upper body, one vertebrae at a time, in a rolling movement to upright position. Lower with a straight back. Repeat.	Contract the core muscles to stabilize the body. Avoid pulling the head backwards at the end of the exercise; stop the movement in neutral position.	Different arm/leg position. The hands unsupported or support on the legs.
Standing. Legs together or hip-width apart. Legs slightly bent. Hands on the back or in front of the legs. Contract the core muscles to stabilize. Keep the back straight. Lower, lean, the torso forward to approx. horizontal position. Return back up (back extension). Repeat.	Contract the core muscles to stabilize the body.	Different arm/leg position. Short or long lever. Arms at sides, by the chest or the head, or above the the head.

EXERCISE	TECHNIQUE

**BACK EXTENSION HOLD
STANDING, ISOMETRIC,
WITH ARMSWING**

Primary muscles:
Erector spinae,
transversus abdominis,
multifidii

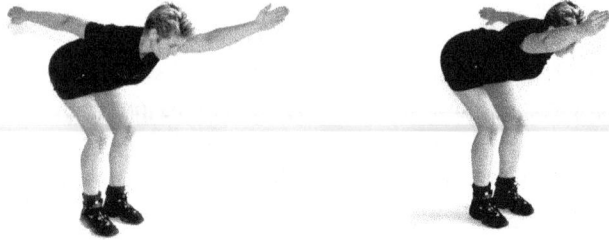

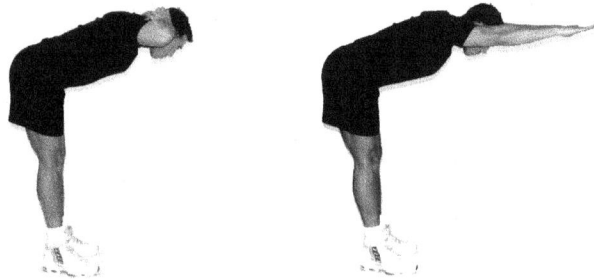

**BACK EXTENSION STANDING
WITH ARM MOVEMENT**

Primary muscles:
Erector spinae,
transverses abdominis,
multifidii

**BACK EXTENSION STANDING
WITH EXERCISE BAND**

Primary muscles:
Erector spinae,
gluteus maximus, hamstrings,
transversus abdominis,
multifidii

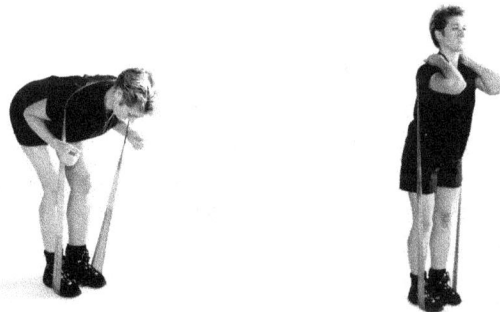

GOOD MORNING

Primary muscles:
Gluteus maximus, hamstrings,
erector spinae,
transversus abdominis,
multifidii

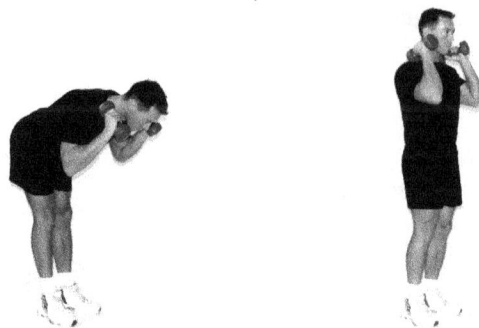

TECHNIQUE	NOTES	VARIATION
Standing. Legs together or hip-width apart and slightly bent. Lean the body forward to approx. horizontal position. Hold this position, any number of seconds, while the arms swing back and forth, fast or slow.	Contract the core muscles to stabilize the body. Neck in neutral position. Do not swing the arms (fast or with a large ROM), if the back starts moving or losing stability.	Different arm/leg position.
Standing. Legs together or hip-width apart. The hands support on the back of the head. Contract the core muscles to stabilize the body. Lower the torso to approx. horizontal position. Extend the arms forward. Hold or return. Return to upright position.	For intermediate exercisers. Not recommended for beginners or people with back problems. Contract the core muscles to stabilize the body. Neck in neutral position.	Different arm position. With or without resistance.
Standing. Legs together or hip-width apart with resistance band anchored around the back and under the feet. The hands are by the shoulders keeping the band in place. Lower the torso to approx. horizontal position. Return to upright position. Repeat.	Contract the core muscles to stabilize the body. Neck in neutral position.	Different arm/leg position.
Standing. Legs together or hip-width apart. The hands hold a barbell on the upper back or dumbbells by the shoulders. Contract the core muscles to stabilize the body. Lower the torso to approx. horizontal position. Return to upright position. Repeat.	Controversial exercise. Because of added, external, resistance and long lever. Not recommended for people with back problems. Contract the core muscles to stabilize the body.	Different arm/leg position. Short or long lever. Arms at sides, by the chest or the head, or above the the head.

9 | Ab and Core Exercises

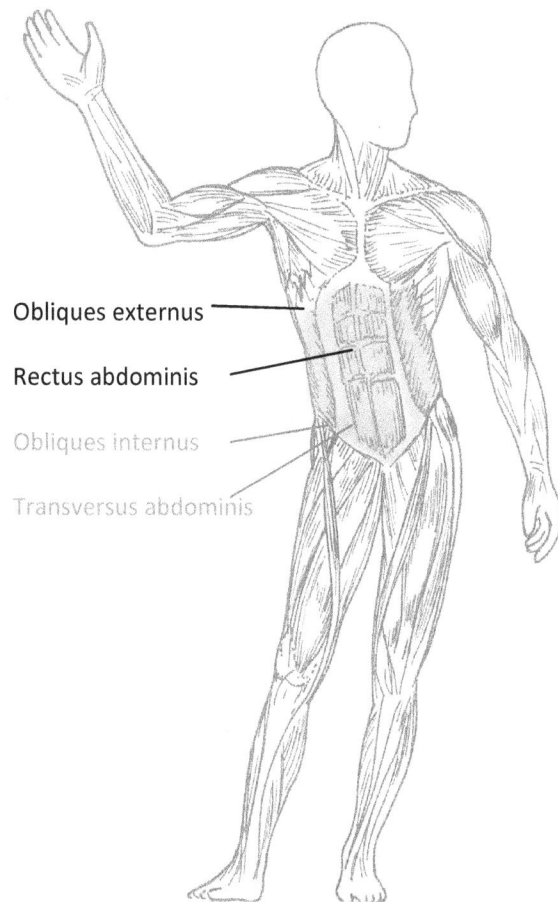

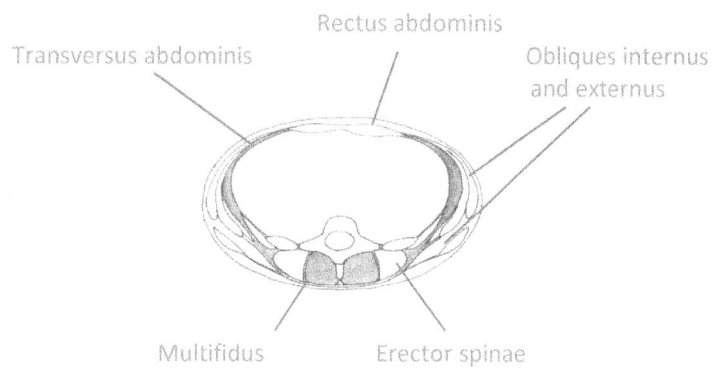

Obliques externus

Rectus abdominis

Obliques internus

Transversus abdominis

Transversus abdominis

Rectus abdominis

Obliques internus
and externus

Multifidus

Erector spinae

EXERCISE	TECHNIQUE

FLATTEN SPINE
SUPINE
BASIC

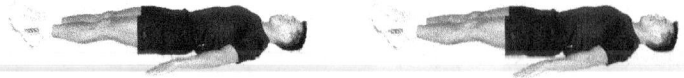

Primary muscles:
Rectus abdominis, obliques
internus and externus,
transversus abdominis

FLATTEN SPINE
SUPINE
EXTENDED

Primary muscles:
Rectus abdominis, obliques
internus and externus,
transversus abdominis

FLATTEN SPINE
SUPINE
LEGS BENT

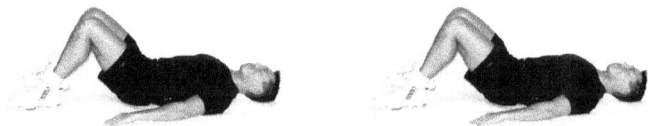

Primary muscles:
Rectus abdominis, obliques
internus and externus,
transversus abdominis

FLATTEN SPINE
SUPINE, LEGS 'TABLETOP',
HIPS AND KNEES FLEXED

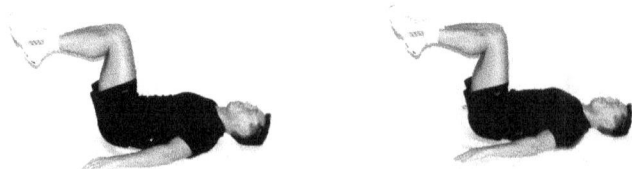

Primary muscles:
Rectus abdominis, obliques,
iliopsoas, transversus
abdominis

Supine. Lying relaxed on the floor. Legs together. Arms at sides. Contract the core muscles. Rectus abdominis flatten the lower back towards the floor and pull ribs and pubic bone towards each other. Hold for 6-10 sec. Release. Repeat 3-6 times.	Basic exercise. Basic training and rehabilitation. Remember to keep breathing. Exercise is called 'flatten spine', but the purpose is to have the lower back in neutral position withour over-arching, hyperlordosis.	Different arm position.
Supine. Lying relaxed on the floor. Legs together. Arms over the head resting on the floor. Contract the core muscles. Rectus abdominis flatten the lower back towards floor and pull ribs and pubic bone towards each other. Hold for 6-10 sec. Release. Repeat 3-6 times.	Basic exercise. Basic training and rehabilitation. Relax the upper body. Remember to keep breathing.	Different arm position.
Supine. Legs bent 45 degrees in the hip and the knees, feet on the floor. Contract the core muscles. Rectus abdominis flatten the lower back towards the floor. Hold contraction for 6-10 sec. Release. Repeat 3-6 times.	Basic exercise. Basic training and rehabilitation. Relax the upper body. Remember to keep breathing.	Different arm position. Different leg position/angle.
Supine. Legs bent 90 degrees at the hips and knees, 'tabletop'. Legs remain in this position. Contract the core muscles. Contract the rectus abdominis to flatten the lower back towards the floor. Hold contraction for 6-10 sec. Release. Repeat 3-6 times.	For intermediate exercisers, who can perform the above exercises. Relax the upper body. Remember to keep breathing, when holding the contraction.	Different arm position.

EXERCISE	TECHNIQUE

**FLATTEN SPINE
SUPINE, LEGS 'TABLETOP',
ONE-LEG**

Primary muscles:
Transversus abdominis,
multifidii, iliopsoas,
rectus femoris

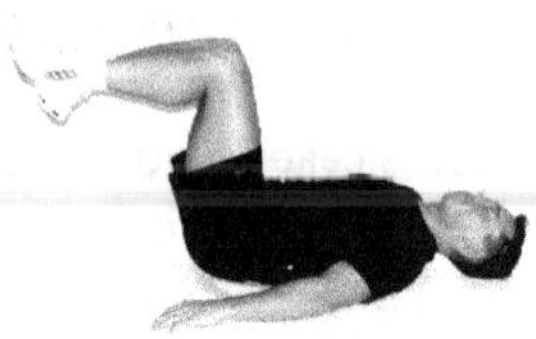

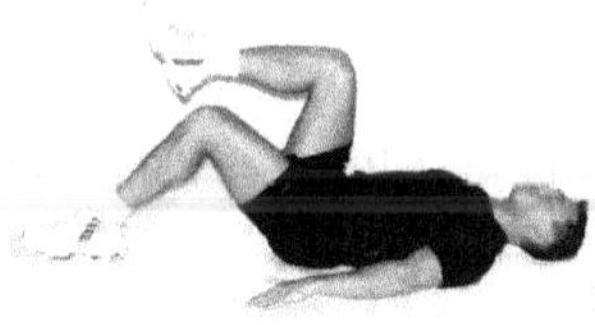

**FLATTEN SPINE
SUPINE, LEGS 'TABLETOP',
BOTH LEGS**

Primary muscles:
Transversus abdominis,
multifidii, iliopsoas,
rectus femoris

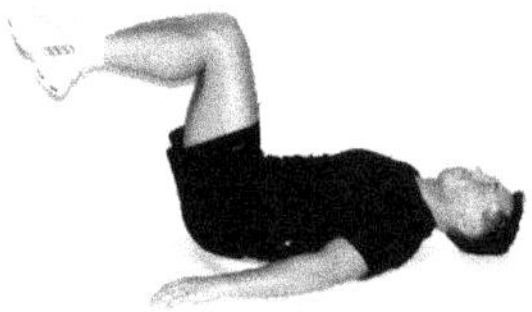

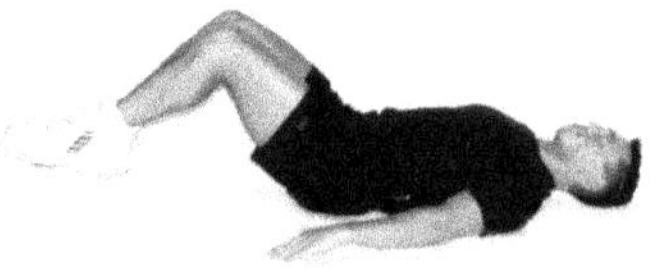

**FLATTEN SPINE
STRAIGHT LEGS
ONE-LEG**

Primary muscles:
Transversus abdominis,
multifidii, iliopsoas,
rectus femoris

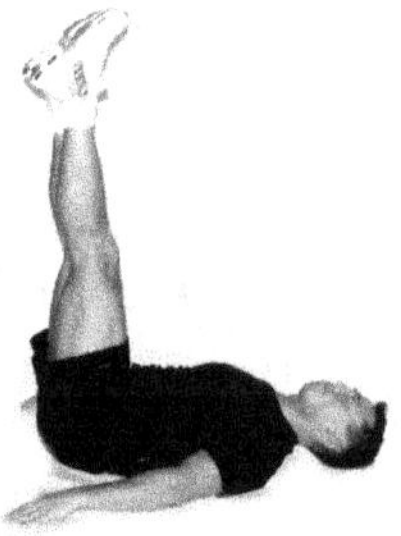

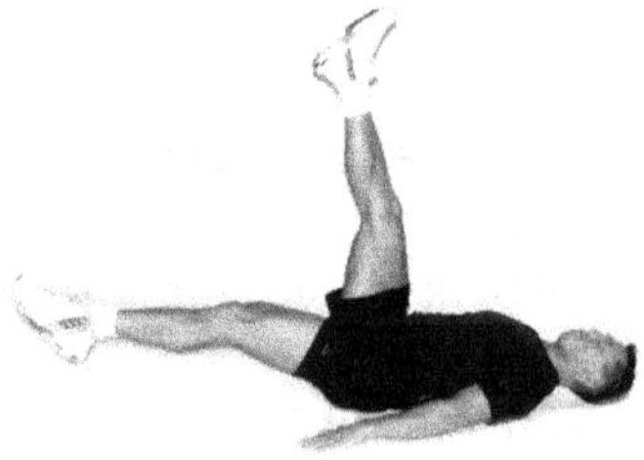

**FLATTEN SPINE
STRAIGHT LEGS
BOTH LEGS**

Primary muscles:
Transversus abdominis,
multifidii, iliopsoas,
rectus femoris

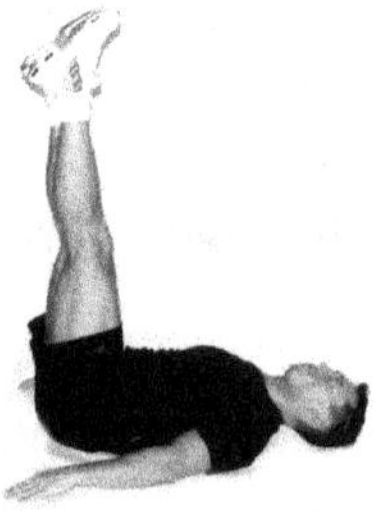

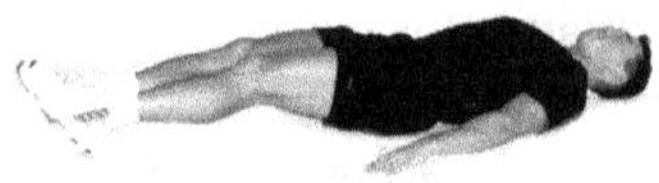

TECHNIQUE	NOTE	VARIATION
Supine. Legs bent 90 degrees at hips and knees, legs lifted. Contract the core muscles. Contract the rectus abdominis to flatten the lower back towards the floor. Lower one leg, touch the foot to the floor, without arching the lower back. Return. Repeat with other leg.	For intermediate to advanced exercisers, who can perform the previous exercises. Remember to keep breathing.	Different arm position.
Supine. Legs bent 90 degrees at the hips and knees, legs lifted off the floor. Contract the core muscles. Contract the rectus abdominis to flatten the lower back towards the floor. Lower both legs, touch the feet to the floor, without arching the lower back. Return. Repeat.	For intermediate to advanced exercisers, who can perform the previous exercises. Remember to keep breathing.	Different arm position.
Supine. Hips bent 90 degrees, knees straight, legs vertical. Contract the ab muscles to flatten the lower back towards the floor. Lower one leg, touch the foot to the floor, without arching the lower back. Return. Repeat with other leg.	For intermediate to advanced exercisers, who can perform the previous exercises without problems. You can put the hands under the buttocks to tilt the pelvis slightly to avoid over-arching. Remember to keep breathing.	Different arm position.
Supine. Hips bent 90 degrees, knees straight, legs vertical. Contract ab muscles to flatten the lower back towards the floor. Lower both legs, touch the feet to the floor, without arching the lower back. Return. Repeat.	For advanced exercisers, who can perform the previous exercises without problems. You can put the hands under the buttocks to tilt the pelvis slightly to avoid over-arching. Remember to keep breathing.	Different arm position.

EXERCISE	TECHNIQUE

TRANSVERSUS EXERCISE

Primary muscles:
Transversus abdominis

PLANK
ON ALL FOORS
KNEES LIFTED OFF FLOOR

Primary muscles:
Transversus abdominis,
multifidii

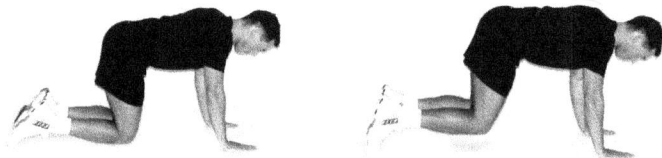

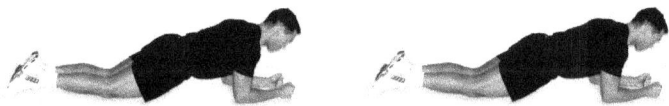

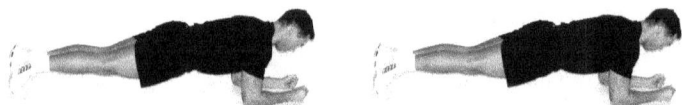

PLANK
FOREARMS AND LOWER LEGS
ON THE FLOOR

Primary muscles:
Transversus abdominis,
multifidii

PLANK
HIPS AND KNEES STRAIGHT
TOES AND FOREAMS ON THE
FLOOR

Primary muscles:
Transversus abdominis,
multifidii

TECHNIQUE	NOTE	VARIATION
Prone. Contract the transversus abdominis. Your abdominal wall flattens and is lifted off the floor. Hold the contraction a couple of seconds. Release. Repeat.	Basic exercise. Remember to keep breathing during the contraction.	Different arm position. Different leg position. Can be performed supine.
On all fours. On the hands. Hips and knees bent 90 degrees. Lift the knees approx. 1 cm off the floor. Contract the abdominal muscles and keep a neutral alignment. Do not arch the lower back. Hold the contraction for up to 1-2 minutes, start with 6-10 sec.	The exercise can be performed at an easier level by keeping the knees on the floor and contrate on working the transversus abdominis. Remember to keep breathing.	Feet can lift one at a time for variation and balance work. **HORSE STANCE.** On all fours. The body contracted. Opposite the hand and the opposite foot lift slightly off the floor, 1 mm-1 cm. Hold for approx. 10 seconds. Change side.
Plank. On the lower legs, hips and knees bent (< 90 degr., eg. 45 degrees). On the hands or forearms. Contract the abdominal muscles. Keep the the lower back in neutral position. Do not arch the back. Hold the contraction for up to 1-2 minutes, start with 6-10 sec.	Basic exercise; provides the foundation for more avanced exercises. Isometric exercise for core stability. Remember to keep breathing.	Different arm/body/leg position. One leg straight backward, liftet from the floor
Plank position. On toes and on forearms or hands. Contract the abdominals. The spine is in neutral position. Do not arch the back. Hold the contraction for up to 1-3 min., start with 6-10 sec.	Intermediate exercise. Isometric exercise for core stability. Remember to keep breathing. Add balance work by lifting one leg or one arm or one arm and the opposite leg.	On the elbows, the hands. On one or both arm(s). Different leg position. On one or both legs. **CROSSLIFT PLANK** On forearms and toes. Lift one arm and the opposite leg. Hold for 15-30 sec. Change side.

EXERCISE	TECHNIQUE

PLANK TURN

Primary muscles:
Transversus abdominis,
multifidii, quadratus lumborum

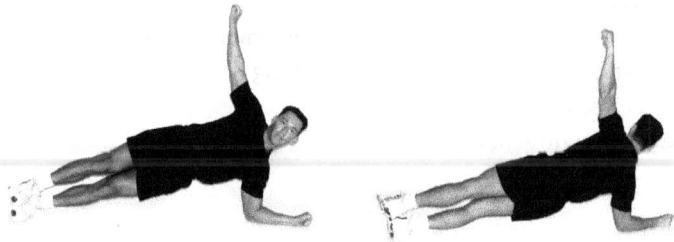

**PLANK LIFT
(ARM OR LEG)**

Primary muscles:
Transversus abdominis,
multifidii, rotators

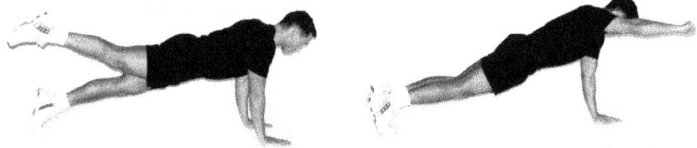

**PLANK CROSSLIFT
ONE-ARM ONE-LEG**

Primary muscles:
Transversus abdominis,
rectus abdominis, rotators,
deltoids, gluteus maximus

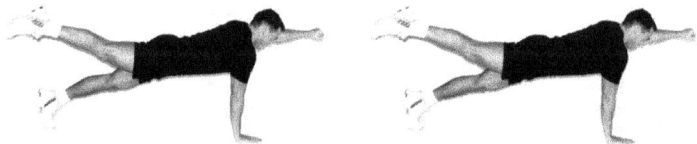

PLANK TRAVELLING

Primary muscles:
Transversus abdominis,
rectus abdominis,
triceps, deltoids

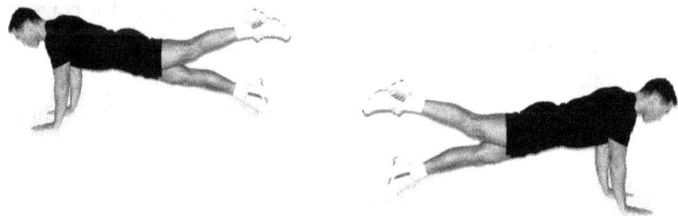

Plank position and side plank position. On toes and forearms. From plank position, turn the body ¼ to side plank position. Turn back to plank. From here turn ¼ to the opposite side, side plank position. Turn back. Hold for as long as desired.	Four phases. Contract the core muscles to stabilize the body. Remember to keep breathing.	Different arm/body/leg position. **TURNING TORSO** Plank position. Hold. Turn ¼. Side plank position. Hold. Lower legs and turn on to the back, support on forearms. Lift into bridge position. Hold. Turn ¼. Side plank. Hold. Return to the start.
Plank position. On the hands (or forearms) and toes. In the plank position lift either one arm or one leg at a time. Lower. Repeat with opposite.	Core training and balance work. Remember to keep breathing.	Different arm/body/leg position.
Plank position. On the hands and toes. Lift one leg and the opposite arm. Hold. Lower. Repeat with opposite.	Core training and balance work. Remember to keep breathing.	Different arm/leg position. **ELBOW TO KNEE** Plank position on one hand and one foot. The free arm and the free leg are pulled towards each other under the body. Return. Repeat with the opposite side.
Plank position. On the hands and toes. Feet remain on the spot. With the arms go for a walk to the right or left, or a full circle. Or: The hands remain on the spot. With the feet go for a walk to the right or the left, or a full circle.	Core training and balance work. Remember to keep breathing.	Different travelling pattern. **PLANK TO THE SIDE** Go for a walk from side to side on the hands and feet.

EXERCISE	TECHNIQUE

**A-FRAME
(PLANK TO A)
PLANK POSITION ON FLOOR**

Primary muscles:
Rectus femoris, obliques
internus and externus,
transversus abdominis

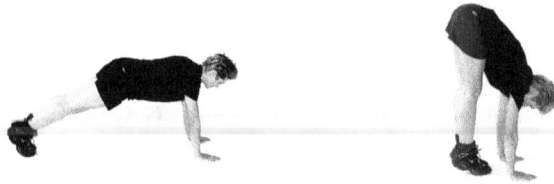

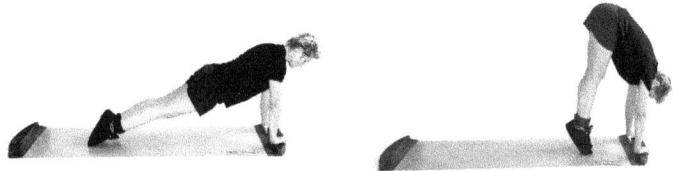

**A-FRAME
(PLANK TO A)
PLANK POSITION ON SLIDE**

Primary muscles:
Rectus femoris, obliques
internus and externus,
transversus abdominis

**DYING BUG
HIPS/KNEES BENT
SUPINE**

Primary muscles:
Transversus abdominis,
multifidii

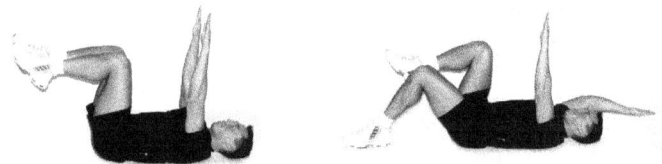

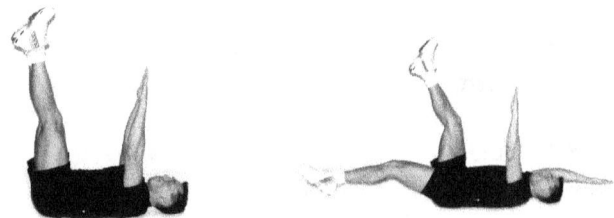

**DYING BUG
HIPS FLEXED/
KNEES STRAIGHT**

Primary muscles:
Transversus abdominis,
multifidii

TECHNIQUE	CHOICE	VARIATION
Plank position. Hands on the floor. Toes on the floor. Body straight in plank position. Contract the abdominals and pull the legs close to the arms. Walk forward with the hands into plank position again – or leg the legs slide backward. Repeat.	For intermediate exercisers. Requires some hamstring flexibility. For strength and stability in the core, shoulders and arms.	On one or both arms. Hop back, hands walk to feet. Contract abs explosively to bring legs forward. **EXPLOSIVE A-FRAME** For very advanced exercisers. From plank contract the ab muscles explosively, propel the body into the air and hands and feet together. Return.
Plank position on a slide. Hands on the endramp. Feet on the slide. Wear shoes and slidesocks Body straight in plank position. Contract the abdominals and pull the legs close to the arms. Let the legs slide backward. Repeat.	For intermediate exercisers. Requires some hamstring flexibility. For strength and stability in the core, shoulders and arms.	
Supine. Hips flexed 90 degrees, knees bent 90 degrees, lower legs horizontal. Arms straight and vertical. Lower one leg, touch foot to the floor without arching the lower back. At the same time lower opposite arm backwards towards the floor. Return with control. Repeat with opposite arm and leg.	For beginning to intermediate exercisers. Contract the core muscles to stabilize the body. Remember to keep breathing.	Different arm position. Different leg position.
Supine. Hips flexed 90 degrees, legs straight and vertical. Arms straight and vertical. Lower one leg, touch foot to the floor without arching the lower back. At the same time lower the opposite arm backwards towards the floor. Return with control. Repeat with opposite arm and leg.	For intermediate exercisers, who can perform the above exercise without problems. Remember to keep breathing.	Different arm position. Different leg position.

EXERCISE	TECHNIQUE

**SPIDER
(STAR SUPPORT)**

Primary muscles:
Transversus abdominis,
multifidii

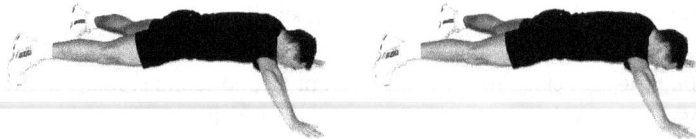

**V OUT
CRUNCH TO V
SUPINE**

Primary muscles:
Rectus abdominis, obliques
internus and externus,
transversus abdominis

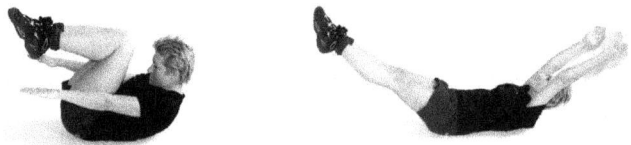

HIP TWIST/LEG CIRCLES

Primary muscles:
Rectus abdominis, obliques
internus and externus,
transversus abdominis,
rectus femoris, iliopsoas

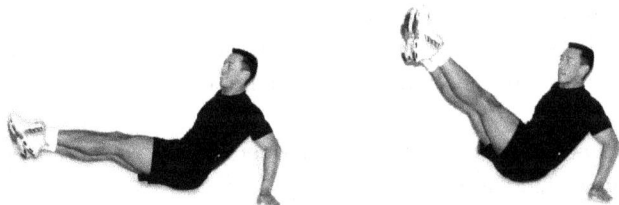

**PLANK
WITH HIP ROTATION**

Primary muscles:
Transversus abdominis,
rectus femoris, iliopsoas,
obliques internus and externus

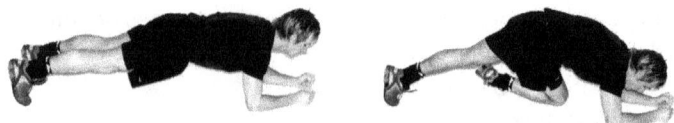

Plank position. On toes and hands. The arms and legs to the side. The arms diagonally forward. The body, spine, in neutral position. Hold.	For advanced exercisers. For core and shoulder stability. Remember to keep breathing.	Different leg/foot positions. On the elbows or hands.
Supine. Hips and knees bent and towards the torso. Arms straight forward. Contract the ab muscles and lift torso and pelvis into a crunch. Extend the arms backwards, 45 degree angle to torso, and lower the straight legs down to a 45 degree angle to the floor: The body forms a V. Repeat.	Contract the core muscles to stabilize the body. Remember to keep breathing.	Different arm position. Different leg position.
Sitting in V-position (V-sit). The bodyweight on the. Legs straight and together. The arms straight, hands on the floor behind the body keeping the body stable. The legs make a circle in the air above the floor. First one way, then the other way.	For advanced exercisers without back problems. Keep the abdominal muscles contracted to protect the lower back. The legs remain together throughout the movement.	Different arm/leg/body position. **CORKSCREW** As leg circles, but with a larger movement finishing on the back- or on the shoulders (like yoga 'plough' with legs straight and together in horizontal above the head. Requires skill and flexibility.
Plank position. On the toes and the elbows or the hands. Contract abdominal muscles. The lower back in neutral. Avoid arching the back. Pull one knee towards the torso and rotate it towards the opposite side. Return. Repeat with the opposite leg.	For core stability and balance work.	Different arm position.

EXERCISE	TECHNIQUE	

**SCISSORS
WITH TORSO ROTATION**

Primary muscles:
Rectus abdominis, obliques
internus and externus,
transversus abdominis

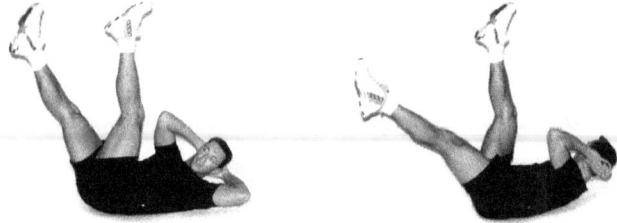

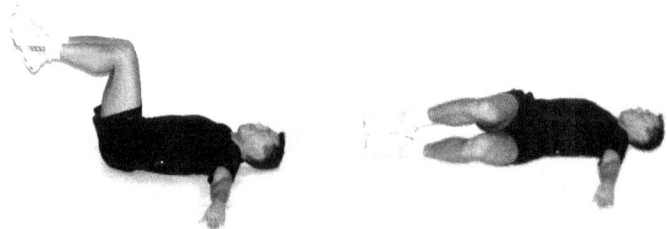

**SCISSORS
(JACKKNIFE OPPOSITE)**

Primary muscles:
Transversus abdominis,
rotators, rectus abdominis,
obliques, iliopsoas, rectus
femoris

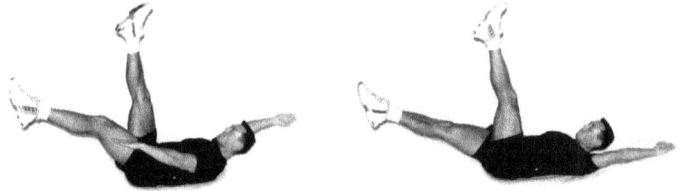

**RAINBOWS
(SUPINE ROTATIONS)
HIPS/KNEES BENT**

Primary muscles:
Obliques internus and
externus, transversus
abdominis

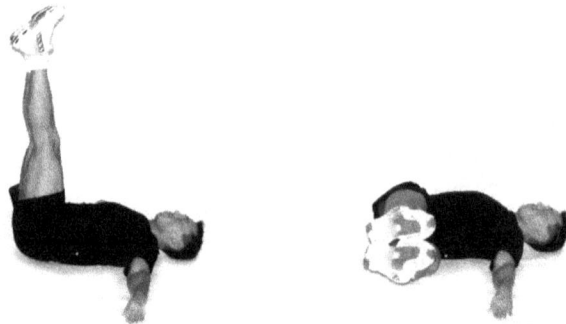

**RAINBOWS
(SUPINE ROTATIONS)
HIPS FLEXED/
KNEES STRAIGHT**

Primary muscles:
Obliques internus and
externus, transversus abd.

Supine. The hands on the floor or the side of the head, elbows out. Legs straight and vertical. Scissor the legs back and forth. At the same time lift and twist the upper body from side to side; rotate towards the top leg.	For advanced exercisers without back problems. Contract the core muscles to stabilize the body. Alternating or to the same side.	Different arm position. Different leg position.
Supine. Abdominals contracted. The arms and legs are straight. Pull right leg up towards the torso, lower left leg. Lower right arm backward to the side of the head, lower left arm down towards the leg. Alternating, right and left, with a controlled movement.	For advanced exercisers without back problems. Control the movement to protect the back.	Different arm position. Different leg position.
Supine. Hips and knees flexed 90 degrees. The arms to the side to stabilize the body. Lower the legs with control to one side, lift, and lower legs to the other side. Repeat.	For intermediate exercisers. Prepare for the exercise by doing the movement with feet on the floor and smaller ROM. Control the movement, avoid 'dropping' the legs, which may overstrain the back. For strength and core stability.	Different arm position. Different leg position. With or without resistance. For beginners. Same exercise, but with the feet in the floor.
Supine. Hips flexed 90 degrees. Legs straight or almost straight. The arms to the side to stabilize the body. Lower the legs with control to one side, lift, lower legs to the other side.	For advanced exercisers. For strength and core stability. Control the movement, avoid 'dropping' the legs, which may harm or overstrain the back.	Different arm position. Different leg position. With or without resistance.

EXERCISE	TECHNIQUE

**AB CURL
LEGS STRAIGHT**

Primary muscles:
Rectus abdominis, obliques
externus and internus

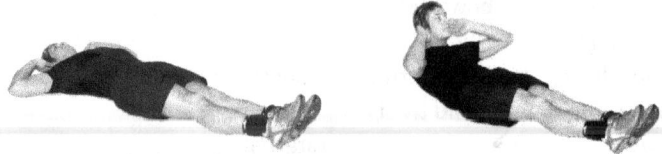

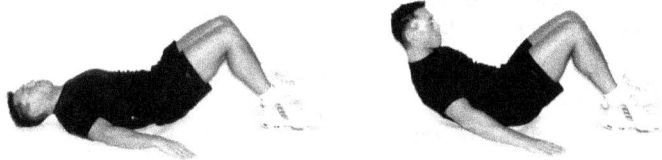

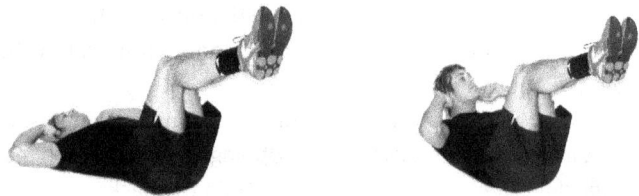

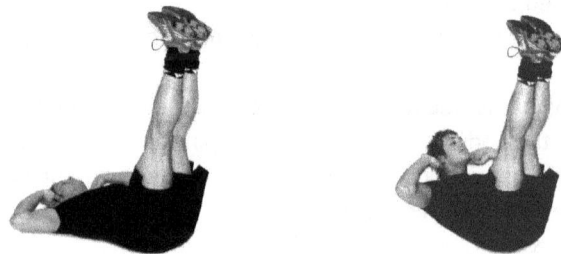

**AB CURL
TRADITIONAL, LEGS BENT**

Primary muscles:
Rectus abdominis, obliques
externus and internus

**AB CURL
HIPS/KNEES
BENT/LIFTED**

Primary muscles:
Rectus abdominis, obliques
externus and internus

**AB CURL
HIPS FLEXED/
KNEES STRAIGHT**

Primary muscles:
Rectus abdominis, obliques
externus and internus

TECHNIQUE	NOTE	VARIATION
Supine. Legs are straight and relaxed on the floor. Contract the abdominal muscles, curl up the torso. Keep the neck in neutral position. Lower.	Not recommended for people with back problems. Legs should not be anchored, as this increase hip flexor activity and may overstrain the lower back). Still the exercise may feel hard or uncomfortable.	Different arm/leg position. The legs can be crossed, if this feels more comfortable. Change leg halfway through the exercise. With or without resistance.
Supine. Feet on the floor together or hip-width apart. Hip and legs bent. Contract the abdominals, curl up the torso. Note: Flexing the ankle, does not change the exercise, but may help some exercisers in stabilizing the body.	Keep the contraction and spine in neutral position: Lower the torso all the way down to touch the shoulder blades and back of the head to the floor, without pausing or releasing. Note: Beginners may find it easier to keep the contraction, if stopping just before shoulder blades touches the floor.	Different arm/leg position. With or without resistance. On floor, bench, ball. **PLATE CRUNCH** Ab curl with a weight plate (or dumbbell, ball or barbell) held on the chest by arms.
Supine. Hip and knees flexed 90 degrees. Lower leg horizontal. Contract the abdominals, curl up the torso. Keep the legs in the same position throughout the exercise. Lower.	It can be hard to keep the thighs vertical – if the legs are pulled a little closer to the torso, the exercise gets easier. Keep the neck in neutral position.	Different arm position. With or without resistance. Auto-resistance: Push both hands hard against the thighs for resistance. With hold: Lift/hold and 1) touch the knees, 2) on the shins, 3) on the foot, 4) lower.
Supine. Hip flexed 90 degrees. Legs must be straight and vertical. Contract the abdominals, curl up the torso. Keep the legs in the same position throughout the exercise. Lower.	Requires some hamstring flexibility. The knees may be slightly bent. Keep the neck in neutral position.	Different arm position. With or without resistance. On floor or bench.

EXERCISE	TECHNIQUE

AB CURL
LEGS BENT/OVER BENCH

Primary muscles:
Rectus abdominis, obliques
externus and internus

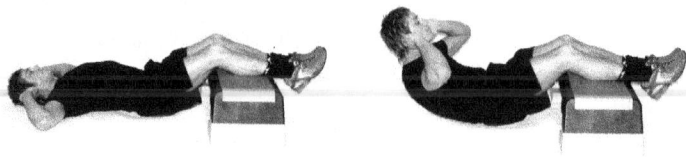

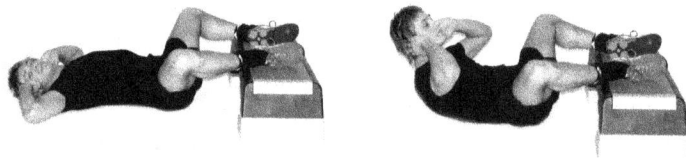

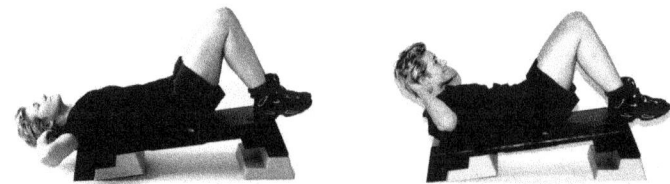

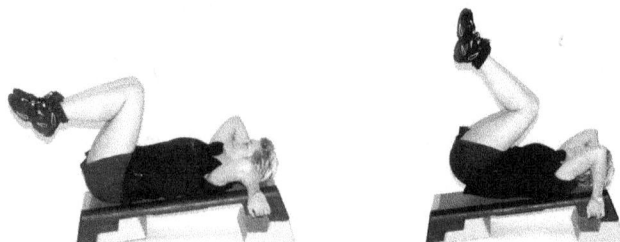

AB CURL
LEGS BENT
LATERALLY ROTATED

Primary muscles:
Rectus abdominis, obliques
externus and internus

DECLINE AB CURL

Primary muscles:
Rectus abdominis, obliques
externus and internus

INCLINE REVERSE AB CURL

Primary muscles:
Rectus abdominis, obliques
externus and internus

TECHNIQUE	NOTE	VARIATION
Supine. Legs resting across a bench. Support hands on the chest or by the head. Curl up the torso. Lower with control.	This position, with the hips bent and the legs resting on a bench, is very comfortable for the lower back.	Different arm position. Different leg position. With or without resistance.
Supine. Legs resting across a bench. The feet close together and the knees to the side. Support hands on the chest or by the head. Curl up the torso. Lower with control.	This exercise minimizes hip flexor activity. Focus is on the abdominal muscles. However, having the legs to the side makes it more difficult to contract the pelvic floor muscles.	Different arm position. With or without resistance. On the floor or legs on a bench.
Supine on a bench. Decline position, the head downwards. Feet together and on the bench. Curl up the torso. Lower with control.	Ab curl in a decline position means the abs must work harder against gravity. The decline position with the head downwards is not recommended for novices or deconditioned exercisers, eg. with high blood pressure or dizziness.	Different arm position. With or without resistance.
Supine on a bench. Incline position, the head upwards. Hands hold the bench in order to stabilize the body. Legs together and vertical or bent and over the torso. Contract the lower part of the rectus abdominis to lift the pelvis and legs from the bench. Lower with control.	Reverse ab curl in an incline position means the abdominal muscles must work harder against gravity to lift the lower body.	Different leg position. With or without resistance.

EXERCISE	TECHNIQUE

**AB CURL DOWN,
(ROLL DOWN)**

Primary muscles:
Rectus abdominis, obliques
externus and internus

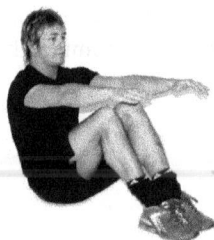

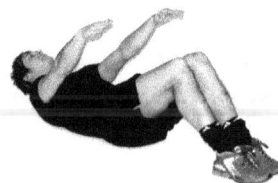

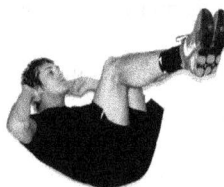

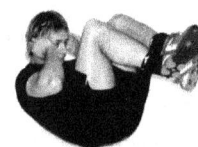

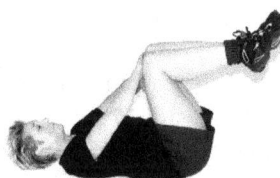

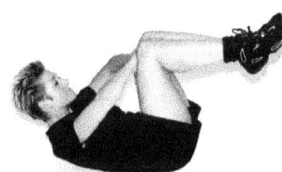

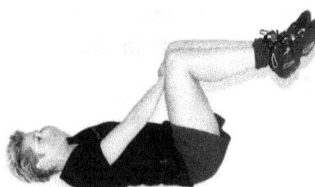

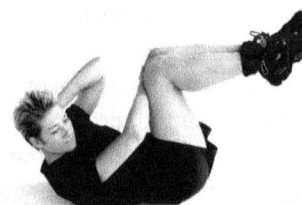

CRUNCHES

Primary muscles:
Rectus abdominis, obliques
externus and internus

**AB CURL
LEGS BENT, 'TABLETOP'**

Primary muscles:
Rectus abdominis, obliques
externus and internus

**AB CURL, WITH TWIST
LEGS BENT, 'TABLETOP'**

Primary muscles:
Rectus abdominis, obliques
externus and internus

Sitting (almost upright). Hips and knees bent. Arms folded on the chest or forward. Tuck tailbone under and roll torso down, one vertebrae at a time. Do not rest, when shoulder blades or back of the head touches the floor, reverse and roll up again. Stop just before upright.	An excellent exercise for abdominal work and lower back mobility. Movement should be in the spine, not the hip. Beginning exercisers may grab hold of the thighs, so the arms may help pulling the torso up past the sticking point.	Different arm position. **ROLLDOWN WITH TWIST** Sitting. Legs bent. The arms straight forward. The torso rolls down and at the same time turns to one side together with the arm of the same side. Roll up again. Repeat to the opposite side.
Supine. Hips and legs bent 90 degrees, tabletop position. Contract the ab muscles to lift the torso and the pelvis at the same time. Lower with control.	Focus on the abdominal work. Be careful not to swing the legs and use the thighs. Focus on both the upper and lower part of the rectus abdominis. Equal focus and force above and below the navel: Think 50 % above, 50 % below.	Different arm position.
Supine. Hips and legs bent 90 degrees, tabletop position. Hands on the thighs. Contract the ab muscles, curl up torso and at the same time press the hands onto the legs to create resistance. Lower with control.	For intermediate exercisers. Contract the core muscles to stabilize the body.	Different leg position. With or without resistance.
Supine. Hips and legs bent 90 degrees, tabletop position. One hand on the thighs. Other hand by the head. Contract the abs and curl and twist the torso diagonally towards the opposite hip. The hand on the thigh presses onto the leg to create resistance. Lower with control.	For intermediate exercisers. Contract the core muscles to stabilize the body.	Different leg positios. With or without resistance.

EXERCISE	TECHNIQUE

KNEE UP
SUPINE

Primary muscles:
Rectus abdominis, obliques
internus and externus,
iliopsoas andrectus femoris

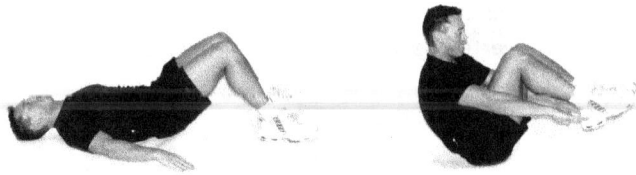

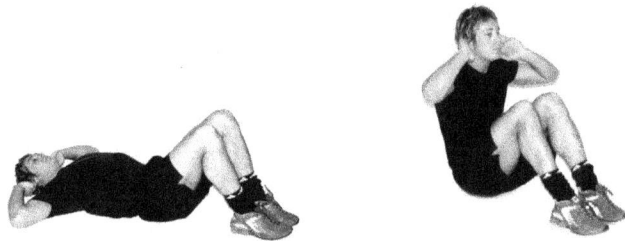

SIT UP
SUPINE

Primary muscles:
Rectus abdominis, obliques
internus and externus,
iliopsoas, rectus femoris

V-SIT
SITTING

Primary muscles:
Rectus abdominis, obliques
internus and externus,
Iliopsoas, rectus femoris,
transversus abdominis

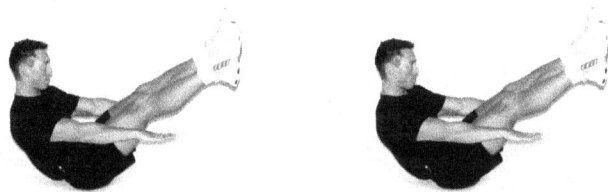

V UP, JACKKNIFE
SUPINE

Primary muscles:
Rectus abdominis, obliques,
iliopsoas, rectus femoris,
transversus abdominis

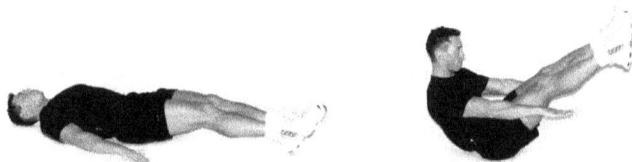

Supine. Arms at sides. Feet on the floor. Hips and knees bent. Contract the abdominals to lift the torso and at the same time flex the hip and pull in the knees, so the body crunches in a sitting knee up position. Lower with control.	For advanced exercisers. Requires some abdominal muscle strength to prevent arching of the lower back. The exercise can be performed sitting on the edge of a bench, with hands either under the buttocks, on the bench or unsupported.	On floor or bench. **KNEE-UP WITH WEIGHT** With dumbbell or bodybar across the ankles. **DIAGONAL KNEE-UP** Pull the legs to the right and left side to involvere the obliques more.
Supine. Legs bent with feet on the floor. Contract the abdominals, curl up the torso and flex the hips to perform a sit-up. Come close to upright position. Lower with control.	For advanced exercisers. Requires some abdominal muscle strength to prevent arching of the lower back. Not recommended for beginners and people with back problems. Past 30 degrees the hip flexors are the prime movers.	Different arm position. Different leg position, straight or bent legs. With or without resistance.
Sitting in a V-sit postion. Legs are together, straight and lifted. Torso and legs is held in a crunch-position, so the body forms a V. Hold the position.	For advanced exercisers. Isometric exercise. For strength, balance and stability. The exercise requires strong abdominal muscles to avoid arching the lower back. Remember to keep breathing.	Different arm/leg position. With bent legs. If needed hold the leg up with the hands on the feet, lower legs or hamstrings.
Supine. Legs are together and straight or slightly bent. Arms are at sides or to the side. Contract the abdominals and hip flexors explosively to curl up the torso and lift the legs at the same time. Hands to the feet or behind the knees. Lower with control.	For advanced exercisers. The exercise requires very strong abdominal muscles to avoid arching the lower back. Train with caution; keep contracting the abdominals to protect the lower back.	Different arm position.

EXERCISE	TECHNIQUE

**OBLIQUE CURL
LEGS STRAIGHT**

Primary muscles:
Obliques internus and
externus, rectus abdominis

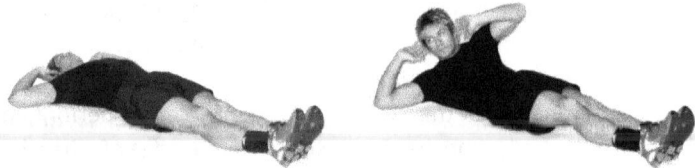

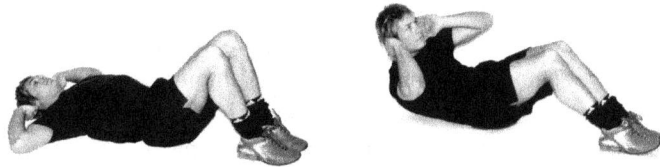

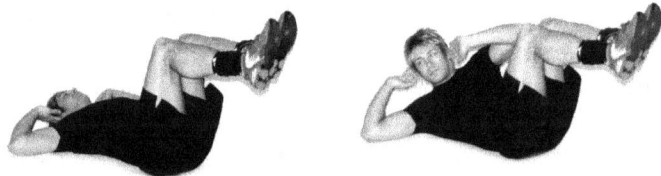

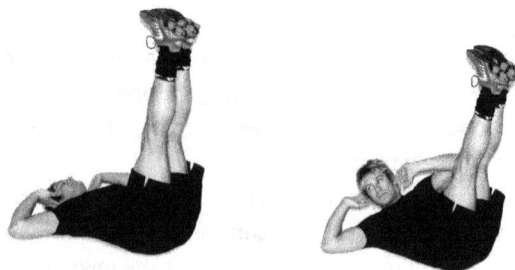

**OBLIQUE CURL
LEGS BENT**

Primary muscles:
Obliques internus and
externus, rectus abdominis

**OBLIQUE CURL
LEGS BENT, 'TABLETOP'**

Primary muscles:
Obliques internus and
externus, rectus abdominis

**OBLIQUE CURL
HIPS BENT/
LEGS STRAIGHT**

Primary muscles:
Obliques internus and
externus, rectus abdominis

Supine. Hip and legs are straight. Contract the abdominals to curl up and rotate diagonally. Lift the shoulder, not elbow, towards the opposite hip. Lift as high as possible to lift the shoulder blades well off the floor. Lower with control.	Avoid rolling from side to side on the shoulder blades. The feet may be crossed, if it feels more comfortable. Contract the core muscles to stabilize the body and keep the lower back in neutral position. Neck in neutral position.	Different arm position. Different leg position. With or without resistance.
Supine. Hips and legs bent. Feet on the floor, optional foot position. Contract the abdominals to curl up and rotate diagonally. Lift the shoulder, not elbow, towards the opposite hip. Lift as high as possible to lift the shoulder blades well off the floor. Lower with control.	Beginners have a tendency to roll from side to side with little activity in the obliques. Initially train one side at a time, change side and repeat. Neck in neutral position.	Different arm position. With or without resistance. On floor, bench or ball. One side at a time or alternating left and right.
Supine. Legs bent, 90 degrees in hips and knees, tabletop position. Contract the abdominals to curl up and rotate diagonally. Lift the shoulder, not elbow, towards the opposite hip. Lift as high as possible to lift the shoulder blades well off the floor. Lower with control.	Avoid rolling from side to side on the shoulder blades. If hands are behind the head: Avoid pulling on the head. Avoid pulling the elbows forward. Keep the elbows back and in the same position during the entire exercise.	Different arm position. On floor or bench. **OBLIQUE CURL WITH RESISTANCE** One hand or forearm press hard against the thighs to create resistance.
Supine. Legs straight and vertical, 90 degree hip flexion. Contract the abdominals to curl up and rotate diagonally. Lift the shoulder, not elbow, towards the opposite hip. Lift as high as possible to lift the shoulder blades well off the floor. Lower with control.	Avoid rolling from side to side on the shoulder blades. If hands are behind the head: Avoid pulling on the head. Avoid pulling the elbows forward. Keep the elbows back and in the same position during the entire exercise.	Different arm position. Different leg position. With or without resistance. On floor or bench.

**SIDETHROW
WITH ARMS AND LEGS**

Primary muscles:
Obliques internus and
externus, rectus abdominis,
transversus abdominis

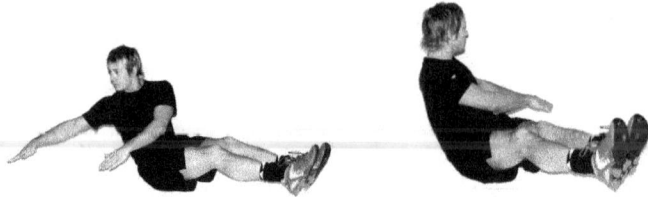

**OBLIQUE CURL
WITH BICEPS ASSISTANCE**

Primary muscles:
Obliques internus and
externus, rectus abdominis,
biceps brachii

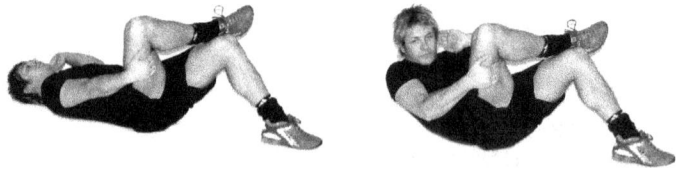

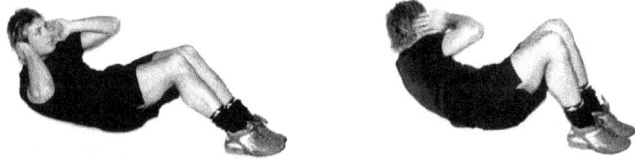

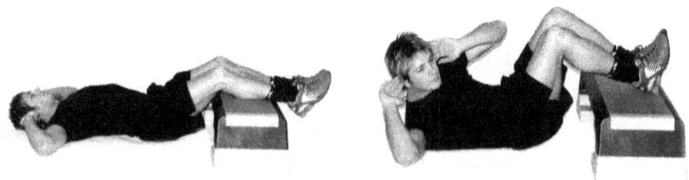

CIRCLE CURL

Primary muscles:
Obliques internus and
externus, rectus abdominis

**OBLIQUE CURL
BENT LEGS OVER BENCH**

Primary muscles:
Obliques internus and
externus, rectus abdominis

Sitting. The arms and leg are straight. The body starts in a V-sit position. Contract the core muscles to stabilize. Move the legs to the right and the arms to the left. Change to the opposite side.	For advanced exercisers. The abdominal muscles should be contracted throughout the exercise to stabilize the body and protect the lower back. Start slowly and gradually increase speed.	Legs straight or (slightly) bent.
Supine. Legs bent. One leg crossed over the other. One hand by the head. The other hand on the top leg. Contract the obliques, curl up, rotate. At the same time contract the biceps to pull the torso up higher than usual. Lower; relax the arm and lower torso with obliquues, no help from arm.	Purpose is to increase the range of motion during oblique curls. Also focus is on the eccentric part of the exercise. A nice variation. Contract the arm as hard as possible to feel a marked contraction in the biceps.	On floor or bench. Both feet on the floor or one leg crossed over the opposite leg.
Supine. Hip and legs are straight or bent. Contract the abdominals to curl and rotate the torso in a circular motion, draw a circle in the air. Start circling from right to left. After a set change direction and circle from left to right.	Shoulder blades are off the floor throughout the exercise.	Different arm position. Different leg position. With or without resistance.
Supine. Legs are across a bench (or feet on the bench). Contract the abs to curl up and rotate diagonally. Lift the shoulder towards the opposite hip. Lift as high as possible to lift the shoulder blades well off the floor. Lower with control. Repeat or alternate.	Avoid rolling from side to side on the shoulder blades. The feet may be crossed, if it feels more comfortable. If so, first set have one leg crossed over the other, next set change legs.	Different arm position. Different leg position. With or without resistance. Same side or alternating.

EXERCISE	TECHNIQUE

SIDE CRUNCH
SIDELYING

Primary muscles:
Obliques internus and
externus, transversus
abdominis

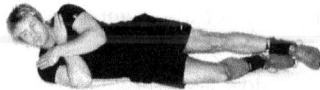

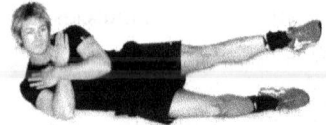

SIDEBEND
WITH CRUNCH
SIDELYING

Primary muscles:
Obliques internus and
externus, rectus abdominis,
transversus abd., multifidii

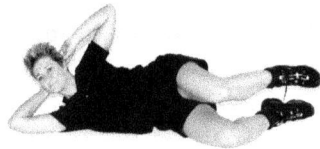

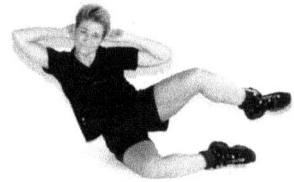

OBLIQUE CURL
LEGS BENT, TO THE SIDES
(LATERALLY ROTATED)

Primary muscles:
Obliques internus and
externus, rectus abdominis

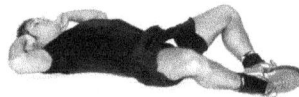

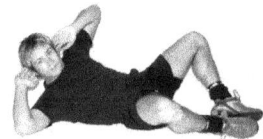

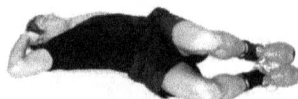

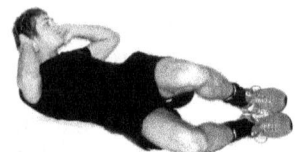

AB CURL
WITH BENT LEGS
TO THE SIDE
SUPINE

Primary muscles:
Obliques internus and
externus, rectus abdominis

Sidelying. Bottom leg is flexed, top leg is straight. Arms are folded on the chest. Perform a sidecrunch, in which the leg lifts sideways towards the torso. Lower with control.	For intermediate exercisers. Requires some skill. Contract the core muscles to stabilize the body. Keep the neck in neutral position (on the photo the head is a bit too high).	Different arm position.
Sidelying. Legs are bent, 45 degrees at the hips and 45 degrees at the knees. The degree of flexion may be changed in order to keep the balance. Perform a sidecrunch and pull the top leg sideways towards the torso. Lower with control.	For advanced exercisers. Requires some skill. Keep the neck in neutral position (on the photo the head is a bit too high).	Different arm/leg position.
Supine. Feet on the floor and together. The knees to the sides. Contract the abdominals to curl and rotate diagonally. Lift the shoulder, not elbow, towards the opposite hip. Lift as high as possible to lift the shoulder blades well off the floor. Lower with control.	Avoid rolling from side to side on the shoulder blades. Avoid pulling on the head, put the hands by the side of the head. Contract the pelvic floor muscles just before curling up.	Different arm position. Different leg position. With or without resistance. On the floor or with legs on a bench.
Supine. Legs are bent, together and lowered to one side. Contract the abdominals to curl straight up, as in a traditional abdominal curl. The legs remain in the same position to the side. Lower with control.	Neck in neutral position. Avoid pulling on the head, put the hands by the side of the head. After a set repeat with the legs to the other side.	Different arm position. Different leg position. With or without resistance.

**CURL DOWN DIAGONAL
SITTING**

Primary muscles:
Rectus abdominis, obliques
internus and externus,
transverses abdominis,
multifidii

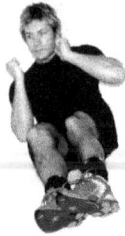

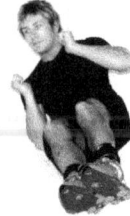

**CURL DOWN (ROLL DOWN)
WITH ROTATION
SITTING**

Primary muscles:
Rectus abdominis,
obliques, transversus
abdominis, multifidii

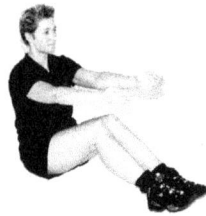

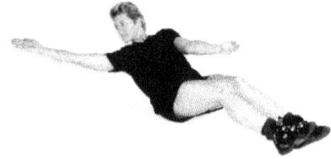

**SIDEBEND
SIDELYING**

Primary muscles:
Obliques internus and externus

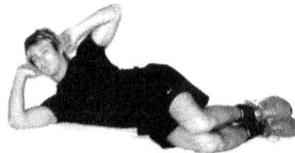

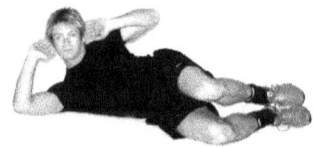

**SIDEBEND
SIDELYING,
LEGS ANCHORED**

Primary muscles:
Quadratus lumborum, obliques
internus and externus

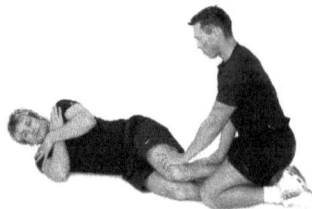

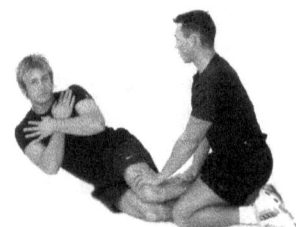

226

Sitting. Hips and knees bent. The body leans to one side, as one unit. Support on one buttock and one heel. Arms are forward. Lower the torso one vertebrae at a time. Do not relax, as the shoulder blades touch the floor, reverse the movement and roll up again.	For intermediate and advanced exercisers. An excellent exercise for back strength and mobility of the lower back. The movement is in the spine, not the hip. Contract the core to stabilize. After a set lean to the other side and repeat.	Different arm position. The arms can be in forward position ready to grip the legs on the way up, if help is needed to get past the sticking point. Or they can be at the chest, by the head or behind the head.
Sitting. Hips flexed and tailbone tucked under. Arms straight forward. Round the back and roll down, one vertebrae at a time. Halfway in the movement turn the body to the side together with the arm at the same side. Return.	Contract the core muscles to stabilize the body. In the pilates version you come all the way forward and extend the hands past the feet. In fitness stop the movement before the body is upright, vertical, to keep working against gravity.	Different arm/leg position.
Sidelying. Legs are slightly bent. Arms are on the chest or by the head. Bend the torso to the side. The shoulders move directly to the side, in the frontal plane. Lift as high as possible. Lower with control.	For increased stability the legs can be crossed, so both feet are resting on the floor.	Different arm position. Different leg position. With or without resistance.
Sidelying. Legs are slightly bent, feet are anchored by a wall bar or a partner. Arms are on the chest. Bend the torso to the side, in the frontal plane. Lift as high as possible. Lower with control.	For lower back strength and stability. Can be performed on a BOSU or ball with the feet anchored under a wall bar.	Different arm position. Different leg position. With or without resistance.

EXERCISE	TECHNIQUE

**SIDEBEND TORSO AND LEGS
(ROCKING), SIDELYING**

Primary muscles:
Obliques internus and
externus, abductors,
adductors, transversus
abdominis, multifidii

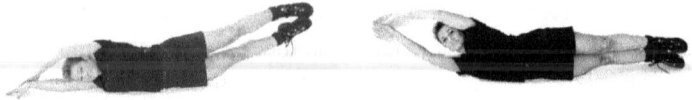

**SIDE PLANK
WITH SIDEBEND**

Primary muscles:
Obliques, quadratus
lumborum, transversus
abdominis, multifidii

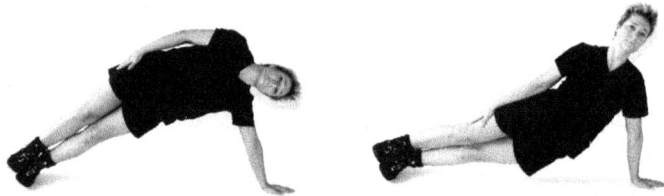

**SIDE PLANK, ISOMETRIC
ONE ARM STABILIZING**

Primary muscles:
Deltoids,
transversus abdominis,
multifidii, quadratus lumborum

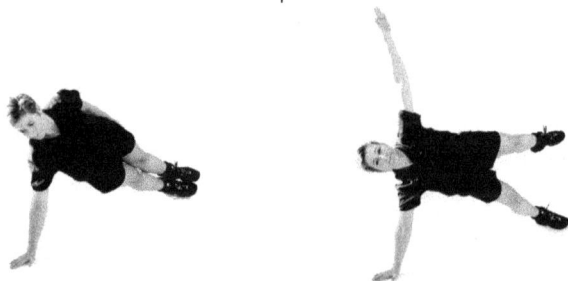

**SIDE PLANK
WITH SIDE A-FRAME**

Primary muscles:
Deltoids, obliques, rectus
abdominis, quadratus
lumborum

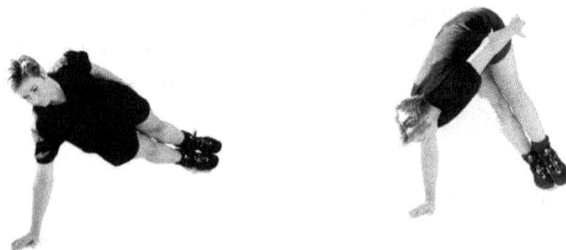

Sidelying. Legs are straight and together. The arms are straight, hands together over the head. Sidebend the torso and lower. Lift the legs up, frontal plane, and lower. Repeat in a smooth continuus movement, rocking from upper to lower body.	For advanced exercisers. For balance, abdominal strenght and core stability. It can be difficult or even uncomfortable perform the rocking movement. Lie on a mat or similar.	Different arm position.
Side plank position. Legs are straight and together. Feet on top of one another or staggered on the floor. Bottom hand on the floor, other arm at the side of body. Lift and lower the body sideways, in the frontal plane.	Contract the core muscles to stabilize the body. The shoulder should be directly over the hand (on left photo the shoulder is working too hard, not an optimal position for this exercise).	Leg/feet i different position. Top arm position is optional. Support on the hand for more balancework. Support on the forearm, longer lever arm, for more strength work.
Side plank position. Legs are straight and together. Feet on top of one another or staggered on the floor. Bottom hand on the floor, top arm at the side of the body. Hold the position. For variation lift and lower the top leg.	For advanced exercisers. For abdominal strength, shoulder stability and balance. Contract the core muscles to stabilize the body.	Dynamic or isometric exercise. Top leg/hip may perform abduction, flexion or extension.
Side plank position. One hand on the floor, other hand at the side of the body. Contract the abdominal muscles, bend the body and pull the legs sidewards towards the torso. Slide the legs back to the starting position.	For advanced exercisers. For abdominal strength, shoulder stability and balance. Contract the core muscles to stabilize the body.	Isometric or dynamic.

EXERCISE	TECHNIQUE

**UNILATERAL ROTATION
(TORSO ROTATION)
ON ALL FOURS
WITH TUBE/BAND**

Primary muscles:
Obliques internus and
externus, rotators, multifidii

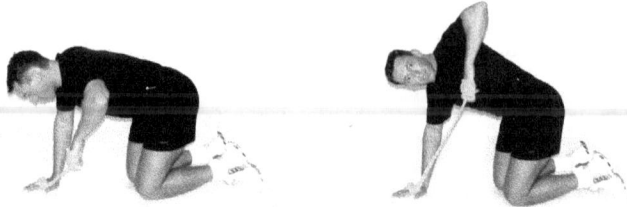

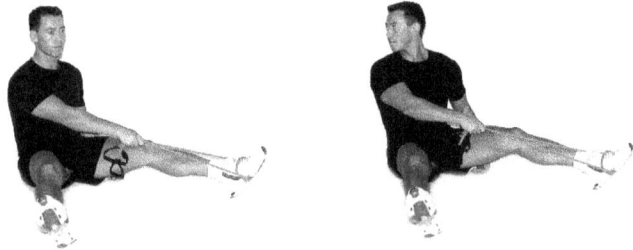

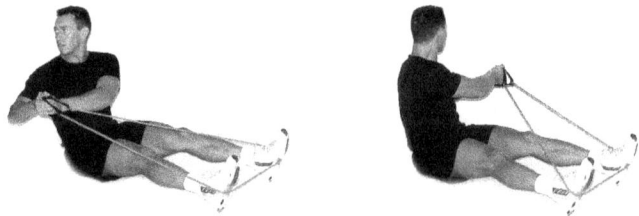

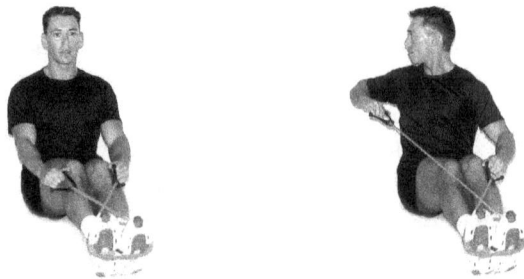

**ROTATION
(TORSO ROTATION)
UNILATERAL,
SITTING WITH TUBE/BAND**

Primary muscles:
Obliques internus and
externus, rotators, multifidii

**ROTATION
(TORSO ROTATION)
SITTING WITH TUBE/BAND**

Primary muscles:
Obliques internus and
externus, rotators, multifidii

**ROTATION
(TORSO ROTATION)
SITTING WITH TUBE/BAND**

Primary muscles:
Obliques internus and
externus, rotators, multifidii

On all fours (three). Band is anchored under one hand, opposite hand holds the other end. Rotate the torso, and the head and neck, to the side of the free arm. Lower with control and repeat. After a set change side.	Contract the core muscles to stabilize the body.	Different leg position. With tube or band.
Sitting. Legs in straddle position. Tube is looped 1-2 times around one foot. Hold the handles with the opposite arm. Arm is straight, passive, throughout the exercise. Rotate torso as far as you can. Return with control. Repeat. After a set repeat with the opposite side.	Contract the core muscles to stabilize the body. Focus on the torso rotation. Concentrate on keeping the torso upright. Focus on the spine as the axis of rotation. The head and neck turn to the side along with the torso.	Sitting on floor/bench/ball. With tube or band. Hold the tubing instead of the handles for more resistance. For additional arm and back work add a rowing movement.
Sitting. Legs in straddle position. Tube under feet. Hands together in front of the chest, with handles in hands. The arms are kept in the same position throughout the exercise. Focus on rotation. Rotate torso as far as you can, return, and rotate to the other side. Return. Repeat.	Contract the core muscles to stabilize the body. Focus on the torso rotation. Concentrate on keeping the torso upright. Focus on the spine as the axis of rotation. The head and neck turn to the side along with the torso.	Sitting on floor/bench/ball. With tube or band.
Sitting. Legs are shoulder-width apart. Tube is looped around the feet with a foot binding. Tube is crossed. Hands hold handles. Rotate the torso to the side, at the same time pull same side arm backwards in a rowing movement. Return. Repeat to the opposite side.	Contract the core muscles to stabilize the body. Focus on the torso rotation. Concentrate on keeping the torso upright. Focus on the spine as the axis of rotation. The head and neck turn to the side along with the torso.	Sitting on floor/bench/ball. With tube or band.

ROTATION, UNILATERAL (TORSO ROTATION) STANDING WITH TUBE/BAND

Primary muscles:
Obliques internus and externus, rotators, multifidii

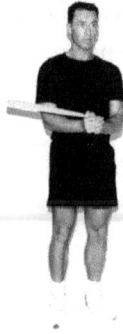

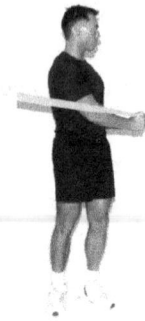

SINGLE ARM PULL WITH ROTATION STANDING WITH TUBE

Primary muscles:
Rotators, posterior deltoid, rhomboids, biceps brachii

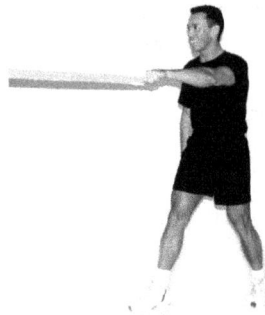

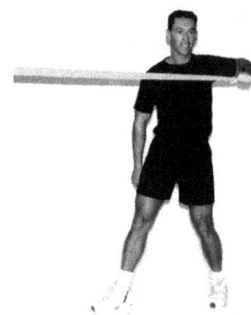

ROTATION WITH ONE-ARM PRESS (SINGLE ARM PUSH) STANDING MED TUBE

Primary muscles:
Obliques internus and externus, pectoralis major, anterior deltoid, triceps brachii

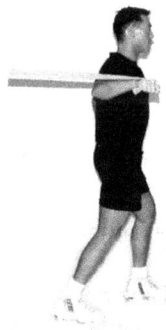

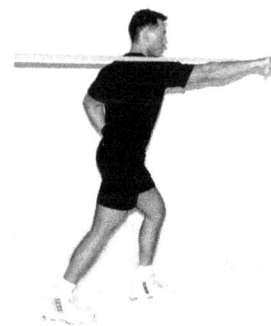

WOOD CHOPS

Primary muscles:
Obliques internus and externus, pectorialis major, latissimus dorsi

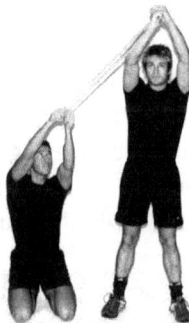

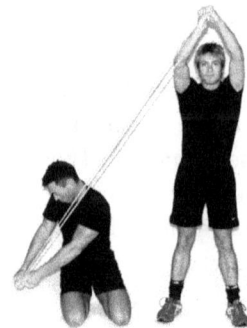

TECHNIQUE	NOTE	VARIATION
Standing. Tube anchored to the side on a wall bar or held by a partner. Hold other end with both hands. Keep arms close to the body and steady. Keep hips neutral and stable. Rotate torso to the side. Return with control. Repeat. After a set repeat to the other side.	Contract the core muscles to stabilize the body. Focus on the torso rotation. Concentrate on keeping the torso upright. Focus on the spine as the axis of rotation. The head and neck turn to the side along with the torso.	Different leg position. Standing, kneeling, sitting. With tube or band.
Standing. Feet are staggered. One hand holds one end of the tube or band. The band is anchored on a wall bar in front of the body. Pull with the arm and then rotate the torso at the end of the movement. Return with control. Repeat. After a set repeat with the other side.	Contract the core muscles to stabilize the body. Focus on the torso rotation. Concentrate on keeping the torso upright. Focus on the spine as the axis of rotation. The head and neck turn to the side along with the torso.	Different arm/the bodys/legposition. Standing or sitting on floor, bench or ball. With tube or band. Turn the head or keep looking forward.
Standing. Feet are staggered. One hand holds one end of the tube or band. The band is anchored on a wall bar behind the body. Push with the arm and then rotate the torso at the end of the movement. Return with control. Repeat. After a set repeat with the other side.	Contract the core muscles to stabilize the body. Focus on the torso rotation. Concentrate on keeping the torso upright. Focus on the spine as the axis of rotation. The head and neck turn to the side along with the torso.	Different arm/body/leg position. Standing or sitting on floor or bench. With tube or band.
Standing or sitting. The hands hold one end of a tube or band anchored high on a wallbar diagonally behind the body (or partner). Pull the arms down and across the body, while rotating the torso. As a 'wood chop'. Return with control. After a set repeat with the other side.	Complex/compound exercise. Can be performed without a partner with the tube or band anchored on a wall bar.	Different leg position.

EXERCISE	TECHNIQUE

**TORSO ROTATION
SITTING**

Primary muscles:
Obliques internus and
externus, rotators, multifidii.

**TORSO ROTATION
STANDING ON ONE LEG**

Primary muscles:
Obliques internus and
externus, rectus abdominis,
transversus abdominis,
multifidii

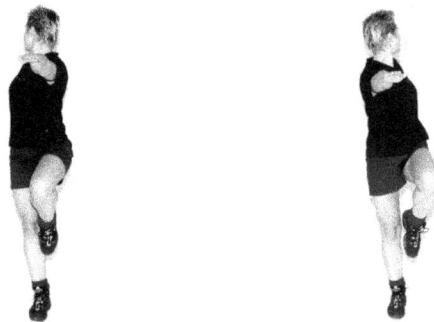

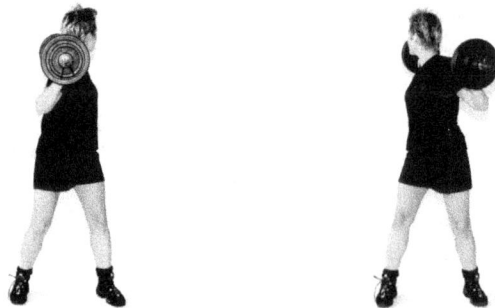

**TWIST WITH BARBELL
STANDING**

Primary muscles:
Obliques internus and
externus, rectus abdominis,
transversus abd., multifidii

JOYSTICK

Primary muscles:
Transversus abdominis,
multifidii, and other muscles

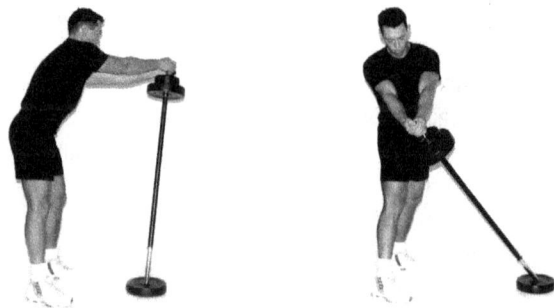

TECHNIQUE	MORE	VARIATION
Sitting. Legs are bent and crossed if needed. Arms are straight to the side a little below shoulderlevel. Rotate the body to one side, rotate as far as possible. Repeat to the opposite side.	Contract the core muscles to stabilize the body. Keep the torso upright; do not rotate with a poor posture.	Different leg position. Sitting on the floor, a bench or an exercise ball.
Standing on one leg. Stand tall with the core muscles contracted. The arms straight to the side a little below shoulderlevel. Rotate the torso to one side, rotate as far as possible. Repeat to the opposite side.	For balance work. Contract the core muscles to stabilize the body. Keep the torso upright; do not rotate with a poor posture.	Standing on one or both legs.
Standing. Legs shoulder-width apart. Contract core muscles. Barbell on the upper back. Keep the torso upright; do not rotate with a poor posture. Rotate the torso from side to side with control, without ballistic uncontrolled action in the torso, hips or legs. Stop. Repeat other side.	For advanced exercisers without back problems. A controversial exercise, which requires control and contraction of the abs, which in the end range of motion have to stop the barbell and reverse the movement. There is a risk of too much torque in the spinal structures.	Different leg position. With or without resistance. With cable pulleys.
Standing. A large weight plate on the floor, one end of the barbell is anchored in the centre. Both hands hold the other end of the barbell. The barbell is moved forcefully in different directions – as a PC joystick – while the core muscles contract to control the movement and keep balance.	For advanced exercisers. Excellent core exercise. Requires skill and strength. Contract the core muscles to stabilize the body.	Different leg position. Combine with lunging movements. Use one arm only. Shift the barbell from hand to hand.

EXERCISE	TECHNIQUE

RUSSIAN TWIST

Primary muscles:
Obliques internus and
externus, rectus abdominis,
transversus abdominis,
multifidii

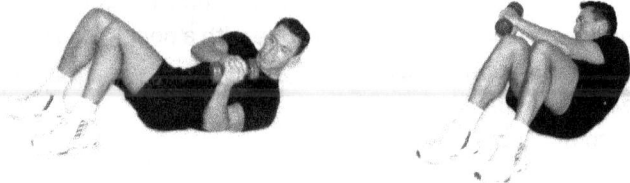

**DOUBLE RUSSIAN TWIST
SUPINE**

Primary muscles:
Obliques internus and
externus, rotators, transversus
abdominis, multifidii

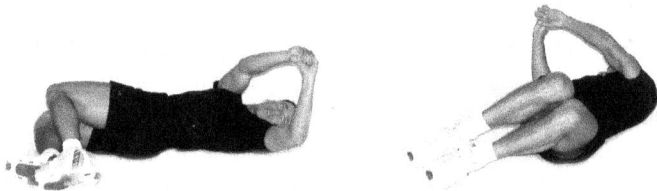

**AB CURL WITH SIDEBEND
SUPINE**

Primary muscles:
Rectus abdominis, obliques,
transversus abdominis

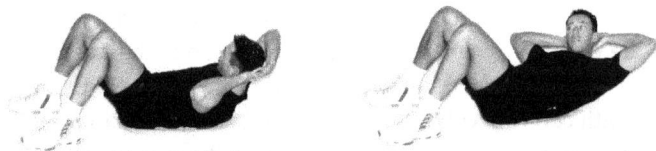

**SIDEBEND HIPS
SUPINE**

Primary muscles:
Rectus abdominis, lower fibres,
obliques internus and
externus, transversus
abdominis,

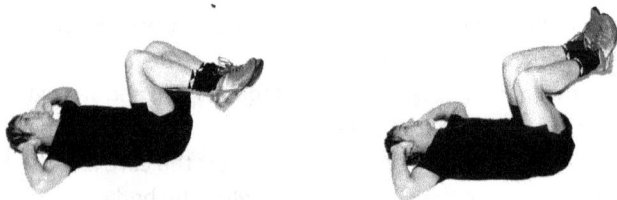

Supine. Hip and legs are bent. Feet on the floor. Hold a dumbbell or weight plate in the hand. The arms are slightly bent. Curl up and rotate the torso from side to side. If possible touch the weight to the floor.	For advanced exercisers. Control the speed of movement. Keep the core muscles and the rectus abdomins contracted during the exercise to protect the lower back.	Different arm position. With a medicine ball, dumbbell or kettlebell in the hands.
Supine. Legs bent and together. Feet on the floor. Hands together and arms vertical above the chest. Curl up and rotate the torso to one side, rotate the legs to the other side. Return with control. Repeat to the opposite side.	Contract the core muscles to stabilize the body.	Different arm position. With a medicine ball, dumbbell or kettlebell in the hands.
Supine. Hip and legs are bent. Feet on the floor, hip-width apart. Curl up and hold this position. Sidebend torso to one side, in the frontal plane; the shoulder towards the hip. Repeat to the opposite side. Lower with control and repeat.	The load is not in the line of pull, however the exercise provides variation.	Different arm position. Different leg position. Lift and sidebend to one side, return and lower. Repeat to the other side. Or lift and hold and sidebend right and left before lowering.
Supine. Hips and legs are bent 90 degr. The legs are lifted, 'tabletop'. Contract the core to stabilize. Keep the torso on the floor. Conctract the abdominals and lift the pelvis up and sidewards towards the torso, in frontal plane. Return. Repeat to the opposite side.	The movement is quite small. Relax the upper body. Keep breathing.	Different arm position.

SIDE PLANK
SHORT OR LONG LEVER

Primary muscles:
Obliques internus and
externus, transversus
abdominis,
quadratus lumborum

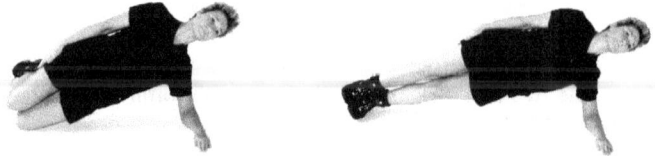

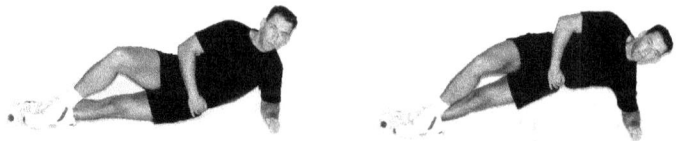

SIDE PLANK
SHORT LEVER

Primary muscles:
Obliques internus and
externus, quadratus
lumborum,
transversus abdominis

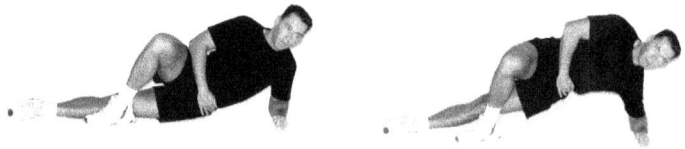

SIDE PLANK
LONG LEVER

Primary muscles:
Obliques internus and
externus, transversus
abdominis,
quadratus lumborum

PILATES SIDE PLANK
WITH EXTENSION

Primary muscles:
Quadratus lumborum,
transversus abdominis,
deltoids

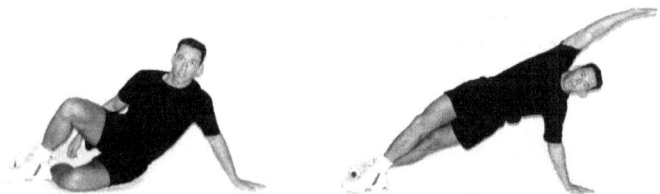

Side plank position. Hips are straight, knees are bent, lower legs on the floor. (Or extend knees to support on side of feet, right photo). The bottom arm is bent and forearm is on the floor. Hold the position.	Isometric exercise. Remember to keep breathing. Keep the elbow below the shoulder. Support on the hand instead of the forearm. The exercise then becomes easier, shorter lever arm, but it becomes more difficult to keep the balance.	Different arm position. Different leg position. **SIDE PLANK WITH ROTATION** In the top position: Rotate the body upwards towards the ceiling or downwards towards the floor.
Side plank position. Support on the forearm. Bottom leg is straight, top leg bent and foot on the floor in front of the opposite knee (of the lower leg). Lift the hip off the floor as high as possible. Hold the position or repeat, lift and lower.	For core conditioning and balance work. Support on the hand instead of the forearm. The exercise then becomes easier, shorter lever arm, but it becomes more difficult to keep the balance.	Isometric or dynamic. Different arm/body movement.
Side plank position. Support on the forearm. Bottom leg is straight, top leg is slightly bent with the foot on the floor in front of the foot behind. Lift hips sidewards up into side plank position. Hold or lower with control.	For advanced exercisers. For core conditioning and balance work. Support on the hand instead of the forearm. The exercise then becomes easier, shorter lever arm, but it becomes more difficult to keep the balance.	Isometric or dynamic.
Sidelying. Support on the bottom hand. The other hand on the knee or by the side. Hips and knees bent approx. 45 degr. Top foot on the floor, in front of the ankle of the leg behind. Extend the top leg, bottom leg follows; lift up into a side plank, in frontal plane. Extend arm overhead. Lower.	For advanced exercisers. For core conditioning and balance work.	Isometric or dynamic. Different arm position. **PILATES SIDE PLANK WITH ROTATION** In the top position: Rotate the body upwards towards the ceiling or downwards towards the floor.

**SIDE PLANK
WITH TORSO ROTATION**

Primary muscles:
Quadratus lumborum, obliques
internus and externus,
rotators, transversus
abdominis, multifidii

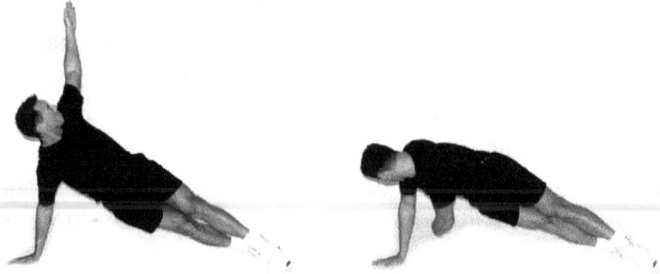

**SIDEBEND
WITH DUMBBELL
STANDING**

Primary muscles:
Obliques externus and
internus, quadratus lumborum

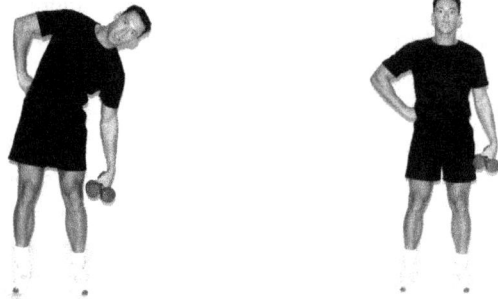

**BICYCLING
SUPINE**

Primary muscles:
Rectus abdominis, obliques
internus and externus,
Iliopsoas, rectus femoris

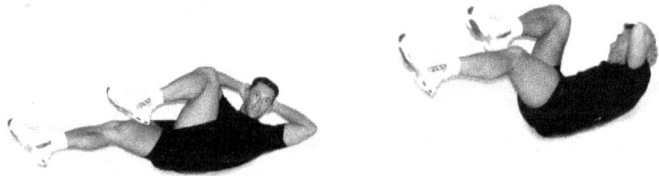

**CAT-CAMEL EXERCISE
ON ALL FOURS**

Primary muscles:
Rectus abdominis and
erector spinae,
transversus abdominis

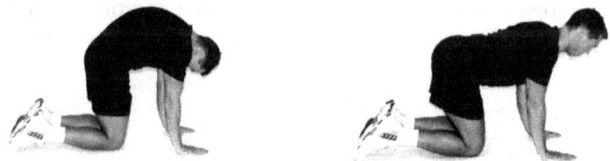

Side plank position. Feet on top of each other or staggered on the floor. Hand or forearm on the floor, directly below the shoulder. Rotate the torso upwards, top arm lifts past vertical. Rotate the torso downwards, the arm moves under the torso. Return to neutral.	For advanced exercisers. For balance and core work. Remember to keep breathing. Contract the core muscles to stabilize the body.	**SIDE PLANK WITH ROTATION FOR INTERMEDIATE EXERCISERS** The legs on the floor. Only the torso is lifted.
Standing. Legs hip-width apart. One the hand on the hip or by the side. The other hand holds a very heavy dumbbell (or a barbell) by the side of the legs. Slowly lower, sidebend, the torso, to the side of the dumbbell. Contract the abdominal muscles and return to upright position.	Only one dumbbell in the hand opposite the working-side muscles. The exercise is less effective with dumbbells in both hands.	Different leg position. With a heavy dumbbell or heavy tube.
Supine. The hands support lightly on the side of the head, elbows to the side. Curl up the torso and twist, rotate from side to side, while the legs are 'cycling' just above the floor. Lift the shoulder towards the opposite hip. Keep the elbows back. Alternate from side to side.	For advanced exercisers. Keep the ab muscles contracted, so the lower back remains on the floor. Avoid over-rotation, and just rolling from side til side on the floor. Lift torso and shoulder towards the opposite hip.	Different leg position/angle.
On all fours. Contract the ab muscles to round the back. Look under the body. Relax. Contract the back extensors and arch the back. The movement is in the lower and upper back, neck is in neutral. Repeat the exercise with slow, continuus movements.	Exercise for mobility and flexibility of the spine and back extensors. A recommended abdominal and back exercise for pregnant exercisers. Can be used as a warm up exercise for stability exercises.	With the hands on floor, bench or ball (small or large). **BREATHING EXERCISE** Inhale deeply through the nose, when sagging the back. Exhale deeply through the nose (or mouth), when arching the back. Inhale for approx. 5 sec. and exhale for 5 sec.

EXERCISE	TECHNIQUE

**POSTERIOR PELVIC TILT
HIP/KNEE STRAIGHT
SUPINE**

Primary muscles:
Rectus abdominis,
focus lower fibres

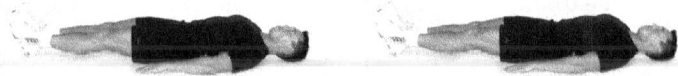

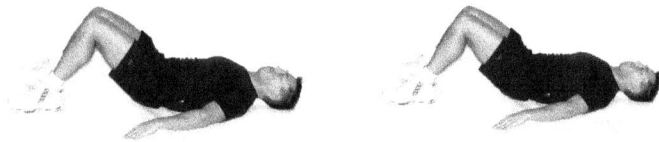

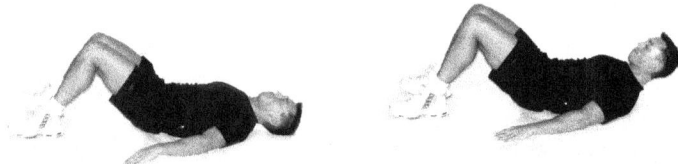

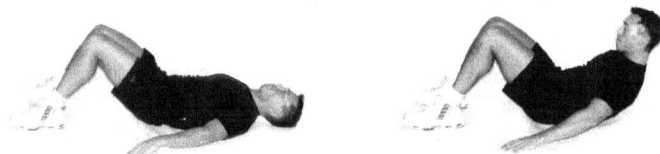

**POSTERIOR PELVIC TILT
HIP/KNEE BENT
SUPINE**

Primary muscles:
Rectus abdominis,
focus lower fibres

**PELVIC TILT
WITH HEAD LIFT
SUPINE**

Primary muscles:
Rectus abdominis,
focus lower fibres

**PELVIC TILT
WITH AB CURL
SUPINE**

Primary muscles:
Rectus abdominis,
focus lower fibres

Supine. Legs are straight and together and on the floor. Contract the lower fibres of the rectus abdominis. Contract the muscles between the pubic bone and the navel and tilt the pelvis posteriorly, hip bones slightly towards the torso. Return to neutral. Repeat.	Basic exercise. For basic training or rehabilitation.	Different arm position.
Supine. Hips and legs are bent, feet are hip-width apart. Contract the lower fibres of the rectus abdominis. Contract the muscles between the pubic bone and the navel and tilt the pelvis posteriorly, hip bones slightly towards the torso. Return. Repeat.	Contract the core muscles to stabilize the body. Relax the buttocks and focus on the abdominal muscles. Avoid contracting the gluteus maximus to initiate hip extension.	Leg/feet in different position, with or without movement. With one or both legs on the floor. On the floor or a bench.
Supine. Hip and legs are bent. Feet are hip-width apart. Contract the lower part of the abs, between the pubic bone and the navel, and tilt the pelvis posteriorly, hip bones slightly towards the torso. Contract the upper part of the abs and lift the head from the floor. Return. Repeat.	Relax the buttocks and focus on the abdominal muscles. Avoid contracting the gluteus maximus to initiate hip extension.	Leg/feet in different position, with or without movement. With one or both legs on the floor. On the floor or a bench.
Supine. Hip and legs are bent. Feet are hip-width apart. Contract the abdominals and curl up the torso and tilt the pelvis at the same time. Torso and pelvis come towards each other. Lower with control. Repeat.	Relax the buttocks and focus on the abdominal muscles. Avoid contracting the gluteus maximus to initiate hip extension.	Leg/feet in different position, with or without movement. With one or both legs on the floor. On the floor or a bench.

EXERCISE	TECHNIQUE

**REVERSE AB CURL
(ABDOMINAL HIP LIFT)
HIPS/KNEES BENT
SUPINE**

Primary muscles:
Obliques internus and
externus, rectus abdominis

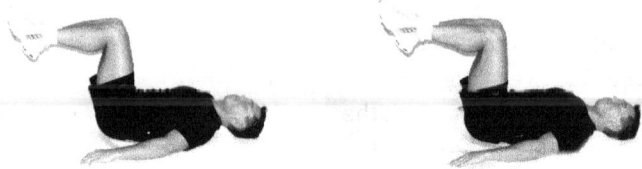

**REVERSE AB CURL
(ABDOMINAL HIP LIFT)
HIPS BENT/KNEES STRAIGHT
SUPINE**

Primary muscles:
Rectus abdominis, obliques
internus and externus

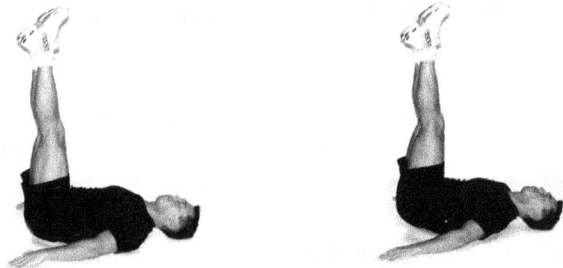

**LEG LIFT
SUPINE**

Primary muscles:
Rectus abdominis, obliques
internus and externus,
iliopsoas, rectus femoris

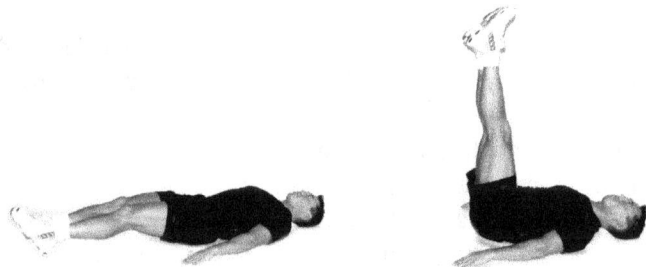

**REVERSE AB CURL
(ABDOMINAL HIP LIFT)
WITH SIDEBEND
SUPINE**

Primary muscles:
Rectus abdominis, lower fibres,
obliques, transverse abdominis

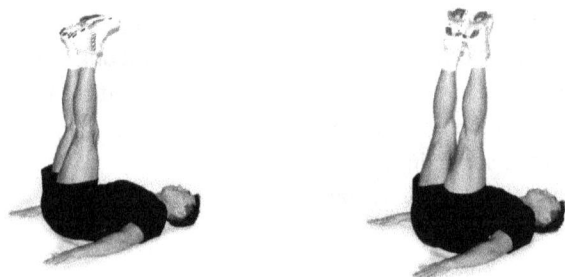

Supine. Hips and legs bent 90 degrees, tabletop position. Contract the lower part of the abdominals, perform a pelvic tilt. The legs are lifted upwards in a straight line. Do not use the hip flexors or swing the legs. Lower with control.	Keep the same angle in the hips and knees thoughout the exercise. Avoid using the hip flexors, so the legs swing back and forth. Keep the legs over the torso to make the exercise easier, shorter lever.	Different arm/leg position. With or without resistance. On floor or bench. Bench position flat or incline.
Supine. Hips bent 90 degrees, knees straight, legs vertical. Contract the lower part of the abdominals, perform a pelvic tilt. The legs are lifted upwards in a straight line. Do not use the hip flexors or swing the legs. Lower with control.	The lumbar spine range of motion is very small, so the hips lift just slightly off the floor. With very strong abdominals you can lift the hips and then the lower back and torso.	Different arm position. Different leg position/angle. With or without resistance. On floor or bench.
Supine. Legs straight and lifted a couple of centimetres off the floor. The arms at sides with the palms on the floor or under buttocks. Contract the abs to keep the lower back in neutral. Hip flexors contract and lift the legs. Stop just before legs are vertical. Lower.	For advanced exercisers. Keep the core and abdominal muscles contracted to avoid arching the lower back. Intermediate exercisers can lift one leg at a time.	Different arm position. Different leg position. With or without resistance. On the floor or a bench.
Supine. Hips flexed 90 degrees, knees straight and legs vertical. Contract the lower part of the abdominals, perform a pelvic tilt, then pull pelvis sidewards towards the torso with the obliques. Return to neutral and repeat to the other side. Lower with control.	In the side bend there is not much work for the obliques as the pull of gravity is downwards, however, sidebending adds variation to the hip lift.	Different arm position. Different leg position. One side at a time: Lift, sidebend, return, lower. Repeat to the opposite side.

10 | Partner Exercises

Exercising with a partner provides more options and makes the workout a sociable experience.

Partner or buddy exercises are a new experience for some exercisers, , which means, however that initially you may have to choose some easier exercises and exercises, where the partners are not too close to each other. In the beginning exercisers may just be sharing a piece of equipment, passing it, supporting it or pulling at either end of it.

To go on to exercising with a partner or friend, hold or support a partner's, shoulder, elbow, forearm or lower legs, or feet against feet. Eventually add exercises holding hands or leaning on or lifting one other.

Focus points:

- Same height and weight – approximately.
- Equal strength – approximately.
- Clear communication between each other.
- Agree upon when to start, so that both are ready.
- Synchronized movements – both work at the same speed.
- A partner initially only support or oppose – later on apply force with control and care.
- Hold or support over or under a joint, never directly on the joint.
- Limit periods, where one partner is inactive. Keep the intensity, so exercise sets, where one partner just assists seem timely and appropriate. Take turns to perform sets, so that no exerciser feels that he or she is wasting time.

One type of partner exercises are traditional exercises, where the partner solely acts as a support or passive partner during the exercise.

'Real' partner exercises are exercises in which a partner is indispensable; eg. exercises with a ball, where you throw or pass a ball to one another, and exercises where the partner resists or assists.

When doing partner exercises it is very important to communicate. Both partners should be observant and focused and both should agree upon when and how to assist or resist.

Never put too much bodyweight into the exercise and be careful not to overstrain any of the joints.

**LATERAL NECK FLEXION
STANDING**

Primary muscles:
Scalene muscles

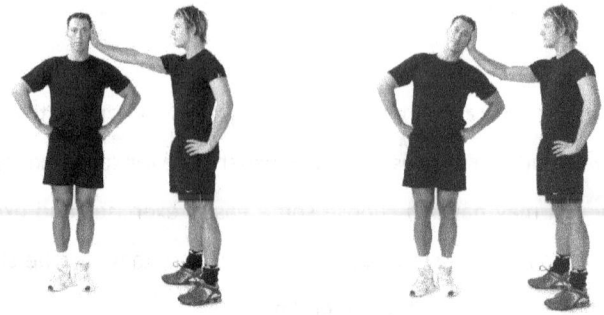

**NECK EXTENSION
ON ALL FOURS**

Primary muscles:
Trapezius, upper part

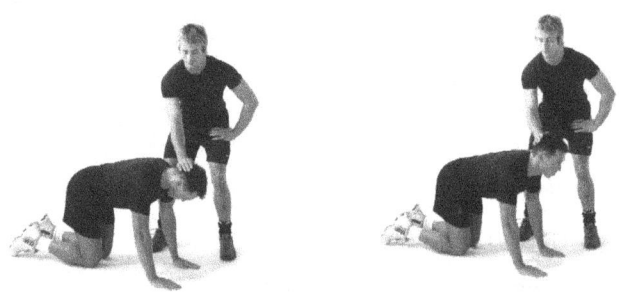

**NECK FLEXION
SUPINE**

Primary muscles:
Sternocleidomastoideus

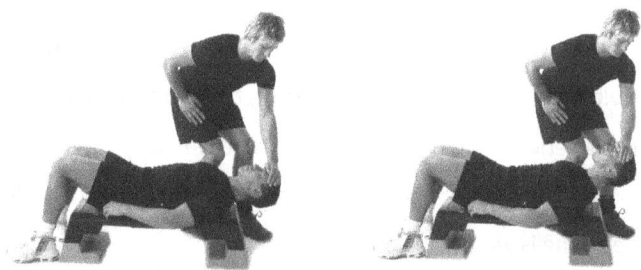

**SHRUGS
KNEELING**

Primary muscles:
Trapezius, upper part,
levator scapulae

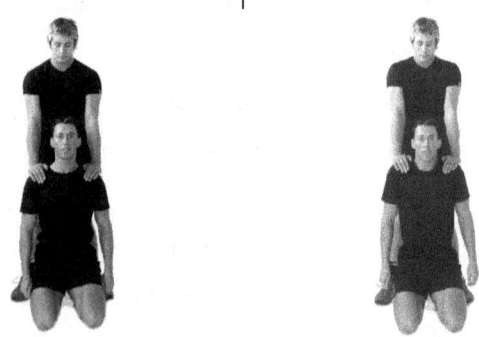

E standing. Body erect and stable. E presses the head sidewards towards the hand of T. (Or: Press the head against own hand providing resistance). Repeat. After a set change side.	Neck exercises: Proceed with caution. The trainer or partner should only hold against, resist the movement with slight pressure, not push or pull too forcefully.	Standing or sitting.
E on all fours. T's hand on the back of the head resisting the movement, while E presses the head backwards into the hand. E resists the movement, while T gently presses the head back to the starting position.	Neck exercises: Proceed with caution. The trainer or partner should only hold against, resist the movement with slight pressure, not push or pull too forcefully.	Different arm position.
E supine on bench. Head/neck is off the bench. T's hand on the forehead of E resists the movement, while E bends the neck/head until the chin touches the chest. T presses lightly on the forehead, while E resists the movement back to the starting position.	Neck exercises: Proceed with caution. The trainer or partner should only hold against, resist the movement with slight pressure, not push or pull too forcefully.	Supine on floor or bench.
E sitting or kneeling. Legs and arms are relaxed. The torso is erect. T support the back of E with the legs and presses down on the shoulders with the hands. E shrugs the shoulders towards the ears and then lowers the shoulders, while resisting the movement.	Neck exercises: Proceed with caution. The trainer or partner should only hold against, resist the movement with slight pressure, not push or pull too forcefully.	Sitting on floor or bench.

EXERCISE	TECHNIQUE

**SIDE LATERAL RAISE
KNEELING**

Primary muscles:
Medial deltoid

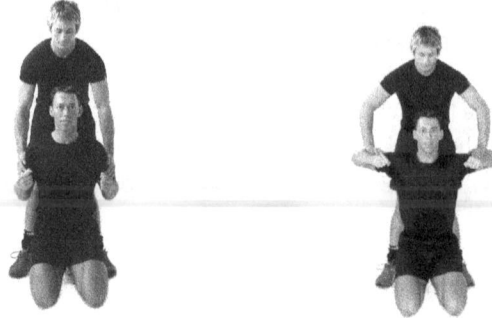

**OVERHEAD PRESS
KNEELING**

Primary muscles:
Anterior and medial deltoid

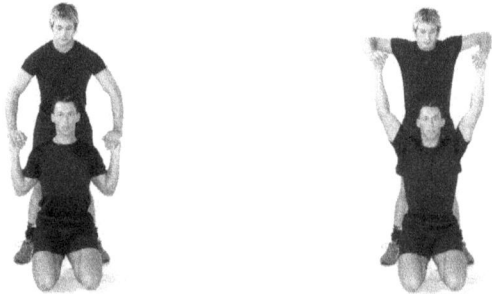

**SHOULDER
MEDIAL ROTATION (IN)
STANDING WITH TUBE**

Primary muscles:
Subscapularis

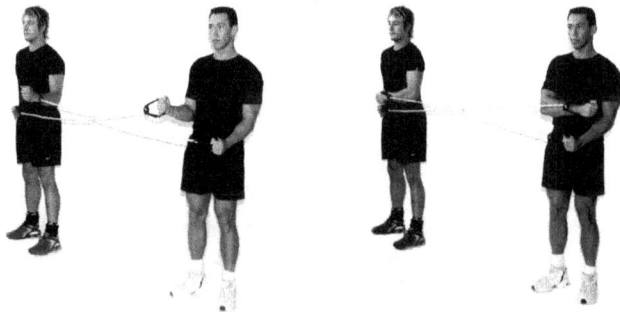

**SHOULDER
LATERAL ROTATION (OUT)
STANDING WITH TUBE**

Primary muscles:
Infraspinatus

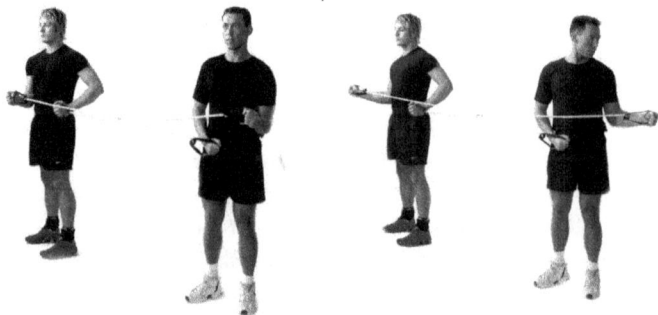

E kneeling. Legs are relaxed. Arms are bent and at sides. The torso is erect. T support the back of E with the legs and presses down on the upper arms of E. E abducts/lifts the arms up/out and then resists the movement, while T pushes the arms downwards.	The trainer or partner provides resistance, but must not push too hard.	Sitting on floor or bench.
E kneeling. Legs are relaxed. Arms are bent, hands by the shoulders. The torso is erect. T support the back of E with the legs and presses the hands down on the fists of E. E presses the arms upwards and then resists the movement, while T pushes the arms downwards.	The trainer or partner provides resistance, but must not push too hard.	Sitting on floor or bench.
E and T standing side by side, both facing forward. Arms bent, upper arms at sides. Tubes are looped around each other. Handles in hands. Outer arm anchors one handle. Inner forearm rotates inwards in front of the body. Return with control. After a set, repeat with the opposite arm.	It is important that both rotate the arm at the same time. Check the tubing for wear and tear before starting.	Different leg position.
E and T standing side by side, both facing forward. Arms bent, upper arms at sides. Tubes are looped around each other. Handles in hands. Inner arm anchors one handle. Outer forearm rotates outwards to the side. Return with control. After a set, repeat with the opposite arm.	It is important that both rotate the arm at the same time. Check the tubing for wear and tear before starting.	Different arm position. Different leg position.

EXERCISE	TECHNIQUE

**PARTNER PUSH-UP
STANDING**

Primary muscles:
Triceps brachii, anterior
deltoid, pectoralis major

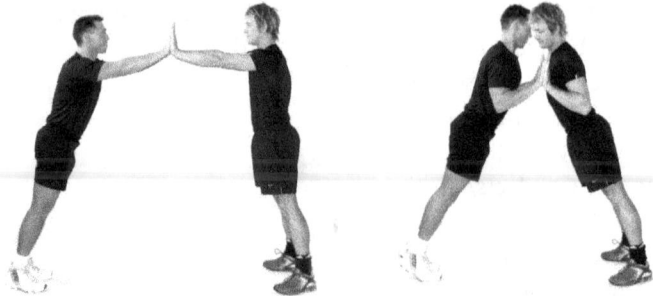

**PUSH-UP
PLANK POSITION**

Primary muscles:
Triceps brachii, deltoids
anterior, pectoralis major

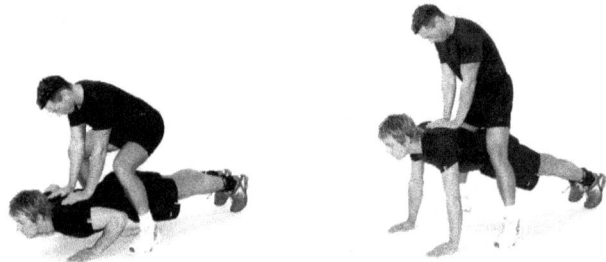

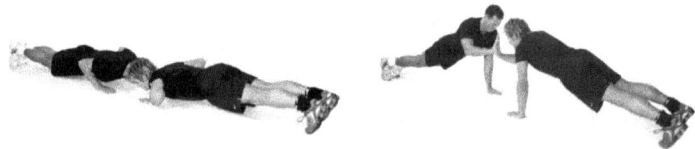

**PARTNER PUSH-UP
WITH CLAP
PLANK POSITION**

Primary muscles:
Triceps brachii, deltoids,
pectoralis major

**PUSH-UP VERTICAL
WITH PARTNER
(PUSHING GEORGIA AWAY)**

Primary muscles:
Deltoids, triceps brachii,
transversus abdominis,
multifdii

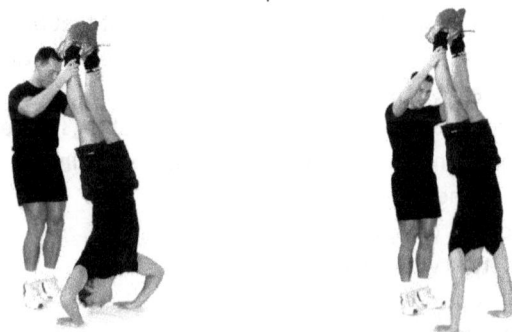

E and T standing facing each other. Palms together. Both partners bend the arms at the same time, so bodies move towards each other. Extend the arms at the same time, so the bodies are pushed back to the starting position.	A standing push-up for balance and coordination. The partners should be of equal height and weight.	Different arm/body/leg position.
E in plank position on the hands and toes. T stands with feet on each side of E's hips with the hands on the shoulder blades. T pushes downwards, while U extends the arms up. T pushes down, while T resists the movement and returns to the starting posiition.	The trainer or partner creates resistance, but must not push too hard.	Different arm/leg position. **ONE-ARM PUSH-UP** The trainer/partner acts as a helper during one-arm push-ups. From the plank position T supports/lifts the torso of E, so the one-arm push-up phase is easier.
E and T in plank position facing each other, 3 feet, 1 m, apart. Both bend the arms, in a push-up, at the same time and extend the arms at the same time. In the top position E and T clap the hand of the partner; both use right arm at the same time. Lower and repeat with opposite hand.	For advanced exercisers. For intermediate exercisers: Perform the push-up on the knees.	Different arm/leg position. Legs together or apart. Arms together (triceps focus) or wide apart (chest focus).
E in a handstand. The hands slightly wider than shoulder-width apart. T holds/supports the lower legs of E. E performs a push-up in the handstand position, focus is on the shoulders. Lower with control.	For advanced and strong exercisers. Excellent core and stability exercise. The partner only supports the legs, he does not provide additional resistance.	With or without partner support.

EXERCISE	TECHNIQUE

BENT ARM CHEST FLYS
SUPINE

Primary muscles:
Pectoralis major,
anterior deltoid

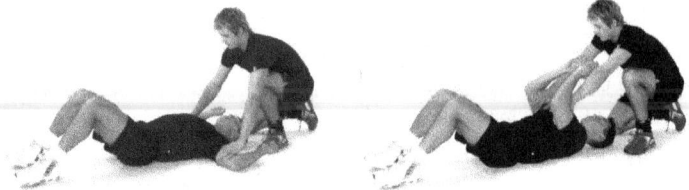

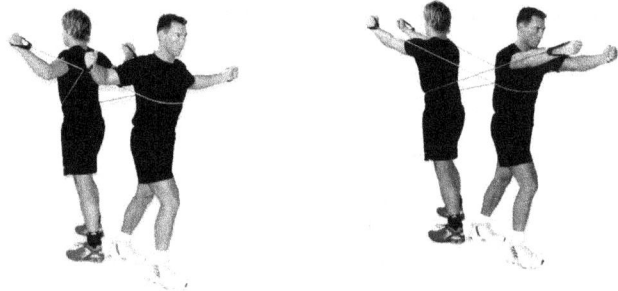

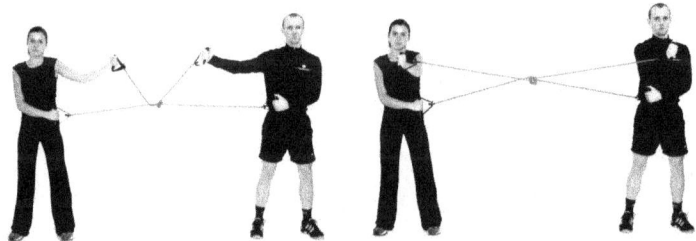

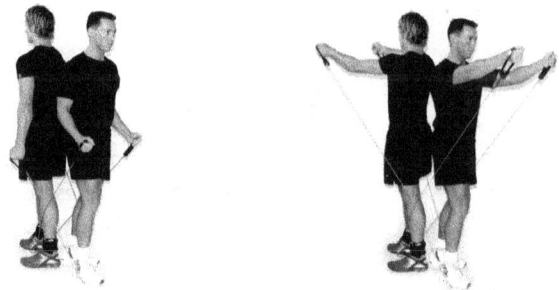

CHEST FLYS
BACK TO BACK WITH TUBE
STANDING

Primary muscles:
Pectoralis major,
anterior deltoid

CHEST FLYS
WITH TUBE/BAND
STANDING

Primary muscles:
Pectoralis major,
anterior deltoid

CHEST PRESS
STANDING, BACK TO BACK
WITH TUBE, LOW ANCHOR

Primary muscles:
Pectoralis major,
anterior deltoid

E supine. The arms are bent 90 degrees and the upper arms are slightly below shoulderheight. T kneels behind the head and pushes against the inside of the upper arms. E adducts the arms in front of the chest. Resist the return movement.	The trainer or partner creates resistance, but must not press too hard. T holds the upper arms just above the elbow, not on the elbow.	Different arm/leg position. On floor or bench.
U and T standing facing away from each other. Tube handles in the hands. Arms slightly bent. Tubes are around the waist or chest of the partners, or looped around each other. Adduct the arms in front of the chest. Resist the return movement.	As the resistance comes from behind and not from the side, the line of pull is not optimal for the fly-movement. Check the tube for wear and tear before using it.	Different arm/leg position. Cross the tubing – instread of putting it around the partner – and adduct the arms at the same time or else the exercise will be too easy.
E and T standing. Side by side. One tube handle in each hand. The outer arm and tube is anchored close to the body. The inner arm is by the side of the torso a little below shoulder level. Adduct the arm in front of chest. Resist the return movement.	The line of pull is from the side giving a more direct pull, than when the tubing is anchored behind body. Is is important that both exercisers adduct the arms at the same time and tempo. Otherwise the exercise does not work.	Different arm/leg position.
E and T standing facing away from each other. One tube handle in each hand. The feet are staggerede and the tube is anchored under the front foot of the partner. Press the arms straight forward and together in front of the chest. Resist the return movement.	Standing with the backs to each other both take a step forward with the right foot and anchor the tubing under the foot and pass the handles to the partner. As the resistance comes from behind and below, not from the side, the line of pull is not optimal for the fly-movement.	Different body/leg position

EXERCISE	TECHNIQUE

**CHEST PRESS
STANDING, BACK TO BACK
WITH TUBE**

Primary muscles:
Pectoralis major,
anterior deltoid,
triceps brachii

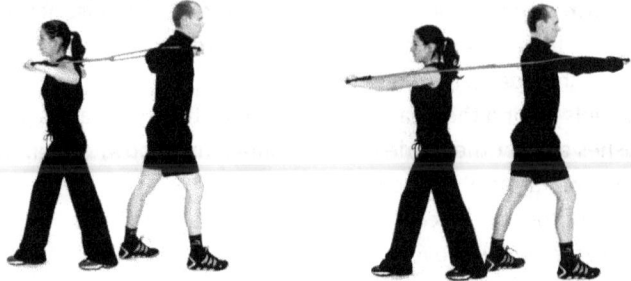

**CHEST PRESS
STANDING WITH LUNGE AND
TORSO ROTATION**

Primary muscles:
Pectoralis major, triceps
brachii, anterior deltoid,
obliques, leg muscles

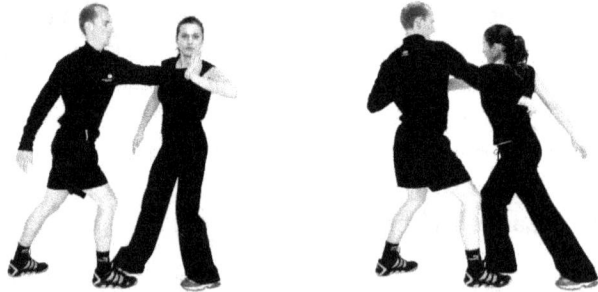

**ROW
STANDING WITH LUNGE AND
TORSO ROTATION**

Primary muscles:
Rhomboids, posterior deltoid,
biceps brachii,
obliques, rotators, leg muscles

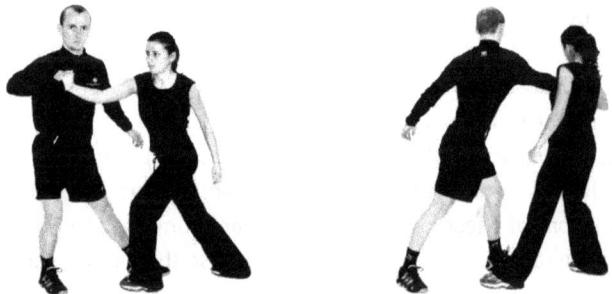

**LAT PULLDOWN
SITTING**

Primary muscles:
Latissimus dorsi,
biceps brachii

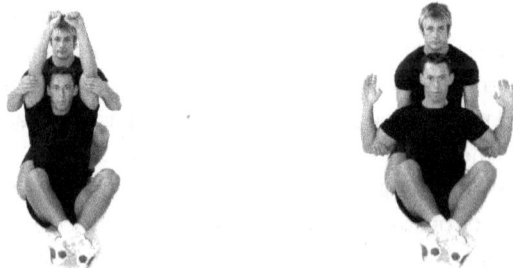

E and T standing facing away from each other. Feet are staggered. A tube handle in each hand. Tubes are looped around each other. Push the arms straight forward and together in front of the chest. Resist the return movement.	Keep the arms at chest level, so the tubing is below the face and the neck. Is is important that both exercisers press the arms forward at the same time and tempo. Otherwise the exercise does not work. Check the tubing before use.	Different body/leg position
E and T standing facing each other. Legs are staggered. Both have left foot in front. Both have their right arm straight forward with palm against that of the partner. E pushes away the hand of T – and rotates torso and shifts body weight to the front leg. T resists. T repeats.	Super partner exercise: Contract the muscles as hard as possible to push and resist. Coordinate the movement force and speed, so both benefit from the exercise. Keep the torso erect, do not lean forward. After a set, change foot and hand.	Progression: 1. Arm/shoulder movement. 2. Add torso rotation. 3. Add lunge forward and back.
E and T standing facing each other. Legs are staggered. Both have left foot in front. Both have right arm straight forward and the hands locked in an 'arm wrestling'- grip. E pulls the arm of T closer – and rotates the torso and shifts the body weight to the back leg. T resists and repeats.	Super partner exercise: Contract the muscles as hard as possible to pull and resist. Coordinate the movement force and speed, so both benefit from the exercise. Keep the torso erect, do not lean forward. After a set, change foot and hand.	Progression: 1. Arm/shoulder movement. 2. Add torso rotation. 3. Add lunge forward and back.
E sitting. The torso is erect. Legs are relaxed. The arms are lifted in the frontal plane. T supports the back of E with the legs and holds the hands under the upper arms of E. E pulls down the arms, while T resists the movement. E moves the arms back up, while resisting the pull of T.	The trainer or partner resists and pulls, but must not pull too hard. T holds the upper arms just above the elbows, not on the elbows.	Sitting on floor or bench.

EXERCISE	TECHNIQUE

**PULLDOWN
BENT ARMS
SITTING**

Primary muscles:
Latissimus dorsi,
posterior deltoid

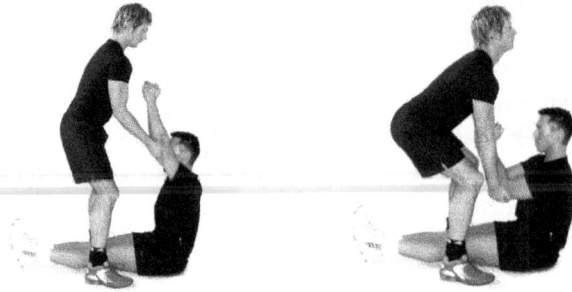

SEATED ROWING

Primary muscles:
Latissimus dorsi,
rhomboids, biceps brachii,
posterior deltoid

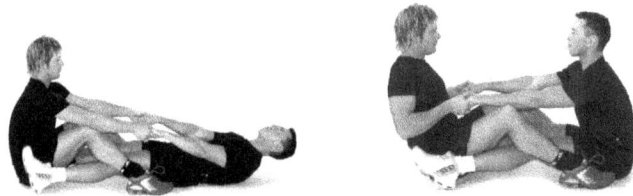

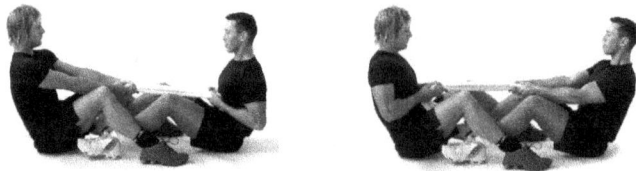

**SEATED ROWING
WITH TOWEL**

Primary muscles:
Latissimus dorsi,
rhomboids, biceps brachii,
posterior deltoid

**LAT PULL
PRONE WITH TUBE**

Primary muscles:
Latissimus dorsi,
biceps brachii

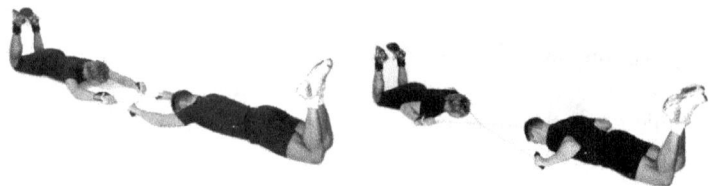

E sitting. Legs are relaxed. Arms are vertical and slightly bent. Elbows forward in the sagittal plane. Torso is erect. T stands facing E, feet on each side of the legs of E. Hands are under the forearms of E. E pulls the arms down, then resist the return movement; T tries to pull E's arms upwards	The trainer or partner creates resistance, but must not push too hard.	Sitting on floor or bench.
E and T sit opposite each other, crossing and locking legs. Hands hold the wrists of the partner. E pulls the hands, and T, towards him. Elbows back in a rowing movement, while T resists. T repeats the movement; T pulls backward, while E resists.	Keep the torso erect to focus on dynamic work for the upper part of the back.	Unilateral, bilateral. Different arm position: Elbows back and along the sides of the torso: Focus latissimus dorsi. Elbows to the side, horizontal plane: Focus rhomboids. Over-, under- or neutral grip.
E and T sitting opposite each other, crossing and locking the legs. E and T each hold one end of a towel. E pulls the towel, and T, towards him. Elbows back in a rowing movement, while T resists. T repeats the movement; T pulls backward, while E resists.	Keep the torso erect to focus on dynamic work for the upper part of the back.	Different arm position: Elbows back and along the sides of the torso: Focus latissimus dorsi. Elbows to the side, horizontal plane: Focus rhomboids.
E and T prone opposite each other, approx. 7 ft, 2 m apart, to be able to extend the arms overhead with tubing outstretched. Tubes are looped around each other. Arms are straight and by the side of the head. E and T pull down the elbows to the sides. Resist return movement.	Check the tubing before use. Keep the heads down. Keep the neck in neutral. The movement is in the frontal plane with arms moving just above the floor.	Prone or kneeling and leaning forward. Either the torso is on the floor or torso is lifted into a back extension, when pulling, but keep the neck neutral, in line with the spine.

EXERCISE	TECHNIQUE

ROWING
WIDE GRIP WITH TUBE/BAND
STANDING

Primary muscles:
Rhomboids, deltoids
posterior, biceps brachii

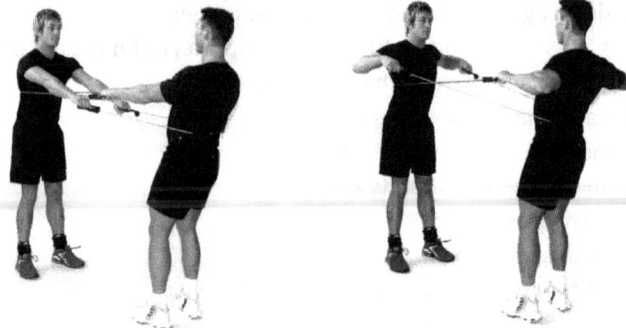

ROWING
NARROW GRIP WITH TUBE
STANDING

Primary muscles:
Latissimus dorsi, deltoids,
posterior, biceps brachii

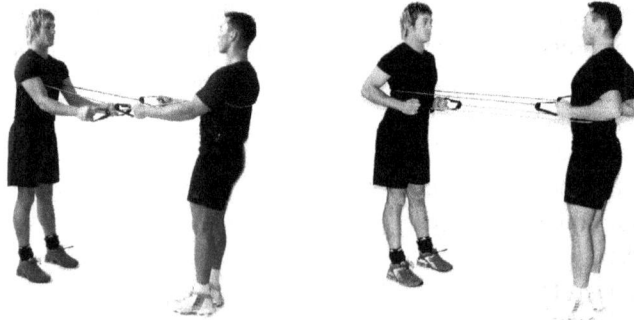

ROWING
NARROW GRIP WITH TUBE
STANDING

Primary muscles:
Latissimus dorsi, posterior
deltoid, biceps brachii

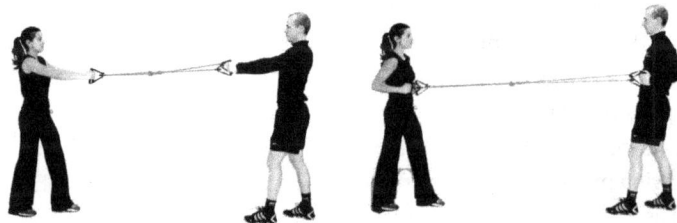

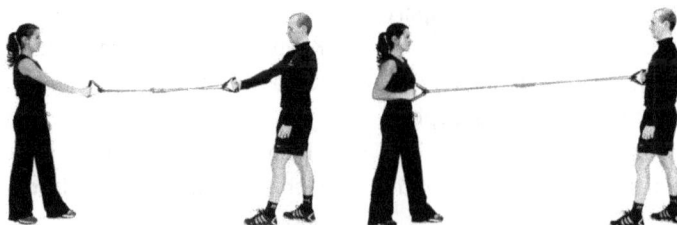

ROWING, UNILATERAL
WITH TUBE/BAND
STANDING

Primary muscles:
Latissimus dorsi, posterior
deltoid, biceps brachii

E and T standing opposite each other. Tubes are anchored behind the back of the partner. Both pull the arms back in a rowing movement, horizontal plane. Elbows to the side at chest level. Resist the return movement.	Contract the core muscles to stabilize the body. Avoid leaning the body backwards (as seen on photo, the partner to the right). Check the tubing before use.	Different leg position. Different arm position: Elbows backwards and along the sides of the torso: Focus latissimus dorsi. Elbows to the side, horizontal plane: Focus rhomboids. Different anchor points
E and T standing opposite each other well apart. Tube is anchored behind the back of the partner. Hands hold the handles. Both pull the arms back in a rowing movement, in the sagittal plane: Elbows backward and along the sides of the torso. Resist the return movement.	Contract the core muscles to stabilize the body. Avoid leaning the body backwards (as seen on photo, the partner to the right). Check the tubing before use.	Different leg positions. Different arm position: Elbows backwards and along the sides of the torso: Focus latissimus dorsi. Elbows to the side, horizontal plane: Focus rhomboids. Different anchor points
E and T standing opposite each other well apart. Tubes are wrapped around each other. Hands hold the handles. Both pull the arms back in a rowing movement, in the sagittal plane: Elbows back past the sides of the torso. Resist the return movement.	Contract the core muscles to stabilize the body. Avoid leaning the body backwards. Is is important that both exercisers pull back the arms at the same time and tempo. Otherwise the exercise does not work.	Different leg positions. Different arm position: Elbows backwards and along the sides of the torso: Focus latissimus dorsi. Elbows to the side, horizontal plane: Focus rhomboids. Different anchor points
E and T standing opposite each other well apart. Tubes are wrapped around each other. One hand holds both handles of own tube. Both pull the arms back in a rowing movement, in sagittal plane: Elbows backward and along the sides of the torso. Resist the return movement.	Contract the core muscles to stabilize the body. Avoid leaning the body backwards. Is is important that both exercisers pull back the arm at the same time and tempo. Otherwise the exercise does not work.	Different leg positions. Different arm positions: Elbows backwards and along the sides of the torso: Focus latissimus dorsi. Elbows to the side, horizontal plane: Focus rhomboids. Different anchor points.

EXERCISE	TECHNIQUE

**LAT PULL
WITH TUBE
STANDING**

Primary muscles:
Latissimus dorsi,
rhomboids, posterior deltoid

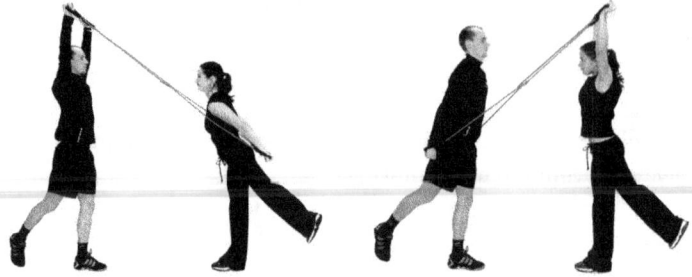

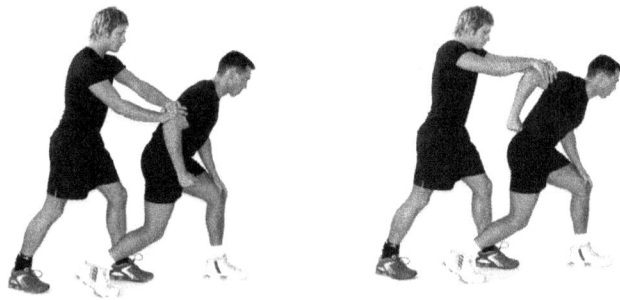

**ROWING, UNILATERAL,
STANDING FORWARD LEAN
(BENT-OVER ROW)**

Primary muscles:
Latissimus dorsi,
posterior deltoid

**BACK FLYS
(REVERSE FLYS)
STANDING**

Primary muscles:
Rhomboids,
posterior deltoid

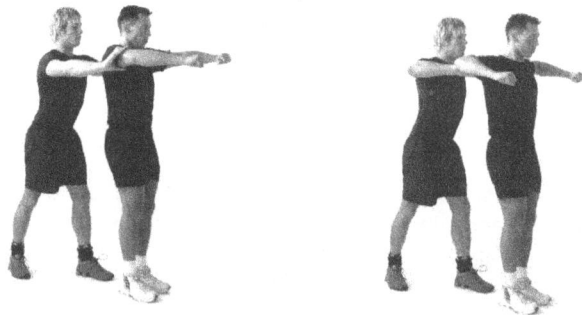

**TRICEPS KICKBACK
STANDING FORWARD LEAN**

Primary muscles:
Triceps brachii

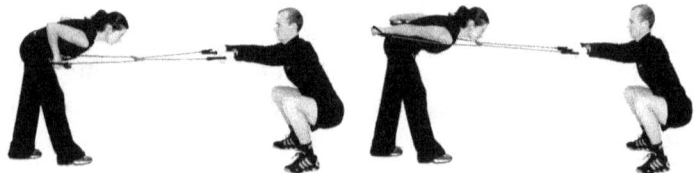

E and T standing opposite each other. Standing on one leg. Tubes are looped around each other. Handles in hands. E pulls the arms upwards, at the same time T pulls downwards. Resist the return movement. Then T pulls upwards and E downwards.	For balance work. Contract the core muscles to stabilize the body. Is is important that both exercisers pull at the same time and tempo. Otherwise the exercise does not work.	Stand on one or both legs. Different arm/leg position.
E standing leaning forward with one hand supported on leg and the other bent 90 degrees and close to the torso. T stands close behind with hands on the upper arm of E. E pulls the arm as far up and back, in the horizontal plane, as possible, while T resists. E resists the return movement.	Keep the back/torso in the same position throughout the exercise.	Different leg position. Sitting or kneeling.
E standing. Upper arms bent 90 degrees and lifted to shoulder level. T stands close behind and hold hands on the back of the upper arms. E pulls the arms as far back, in the horizontal plane, as possible, while T resists. E resists the return movement.	Contract the core muscles to stabilize the body.	Different leg position. Sitting or kneeling.
E standing with legs staggered. Torso leaning forward, 60-80 degrees. T in a squat with arms straight forward. Tubes are looped around each other. Handles in hands. E's upper arms are horizontal, elbows bent. Elbows extend, forearms move in line with upper arms. Resist the return movement.	Contract the core muscles to stabilize the body. Combination exercise in which E and T performs different exercises.	Stand on one or both legs.

EXERCISE	TECHNIQUE

**TRICEPS EXTENSION
KNEELING**

Primary muscles:
Triceps brachii

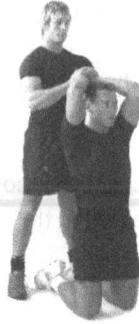

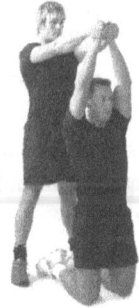

**BICEPS CURL AND
TRICEPS PUSH DOWN
STANDING**

Primary muscles:
Biceps brachii
(triceps brachii)

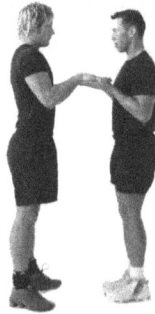

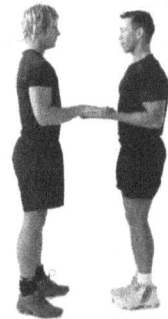

**BICEPS PULL UP
WITH PARTNER**

Primary muscles:
Biceps brachii,
latissimus dorsi

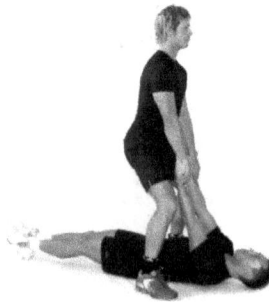

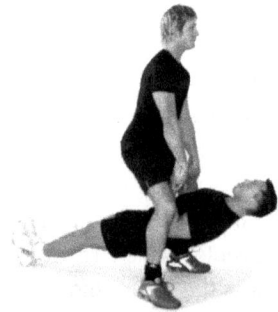

**BOXING PRESSES
STANDING**

Primary muscles:
Pectoralis major, rhomboids,
triceps brachii, biceps brachii

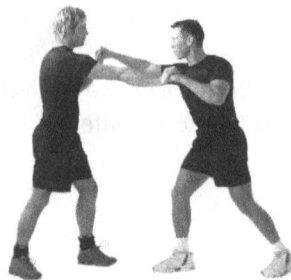

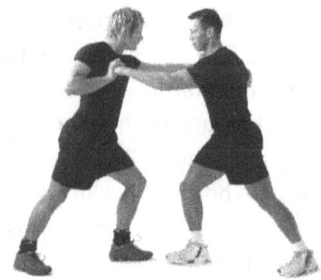

E kneeling. Arms are straight and vertical, hands are together. The torso is erect. T supports the back of E with the legs. T pushes hands down on E's clenched hands. E extends the elbows, arms up, while T resists the movement. E resists the return movement.	The trainer or partner creates resistance, but must not push too hard. Be careful of the elbows in this exercise, do not apply too much pressure.	Sitting on floor or bench.
E standing. One upper arm close to the body. T pushes both hands down into the hand of E. E bends the elbow, arm, while T resists. E resists, while T pushes the arm down.	The trainer or partner creates resistance, but must not press too hard.	Unilateral, bilateral. Different leg position.
E supine. Legs bent or straight. Arms are vertical. Hands hold the wrists of T, underhand grip. T stands astride with the torso erect and the hands around the wrists of E with an overhand grip. E bends the arms to perform a pull-up. Lower with control.	Contract the core muscles to stabilize the body. Pull up with control. It is important that T keeps the torso upright to protect the back. Avoid leaning forward. Legs firmly on the floor and apart. Arms are relaxed.	Different body/leg position. Legs bent or straight (short or long lever). The arms of the exerciser may be crossed. **BICEPS ONE-ARM PULL-UP** Same exercise, but pull up with only one arm.
E and T standing opposite each other. The hands against each other (E's fists may be clenched with T 's hands cupping them). The arms in horizontal plane. E makes a boxing movement with arms alternating, while the partner resists the movement. Change. Repeat.	The trainer or partner creates resistance, but must not push too hard. Avoid forcing limb joints into awkward positions.	Different body/leg position.

**SQUAT
HOLDING HANDS
STANDING**

Primary muscles:
Quadriceps,
gluteus maximus, hamstrings

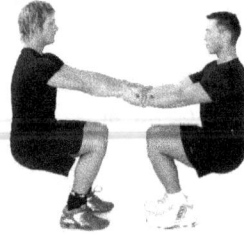

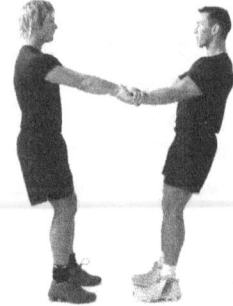

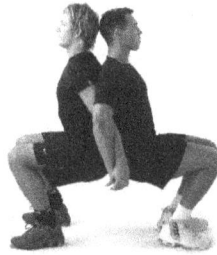

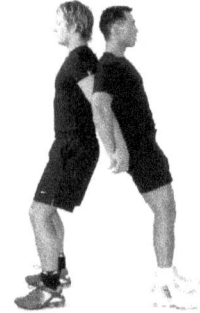

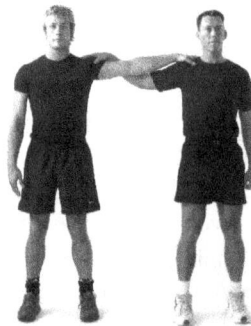

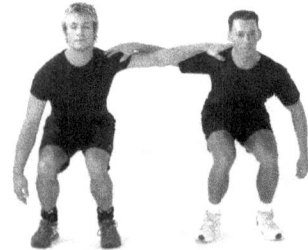

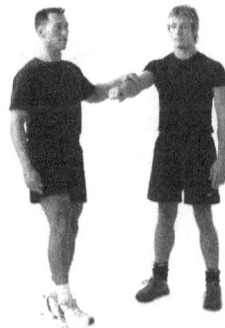

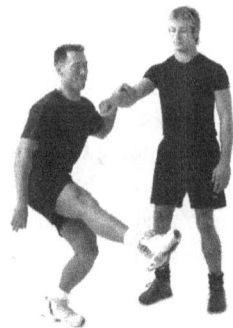

**SQUAT
STANDING, BACK TO BACK**

Primary muscles:
Quadriceps,
gluteus maximus, hamstrings

**SQUAT
STANDING, SIDE BY SIDE**

Primary muscles:
Quadriceps,
gluteus maximus, hamstrings

**ONE-LEG SQUAT
(SINGLE LEG SQUAT)
STANDING WITH SUPPORT**

Primary muscles:
Quadriceps,
gluteus maximus, hamstrings

E and T standing opposite each other. Holding hands or wrists Legs are shoulder-width apart. Toes just opposite those of the partner. Bend the legs to parallel squat or deeper. Return to the starting position without pausing.	For this exercise E and T should be of approximately the same height and weight. E and T must bend the legs at the same time.	Different body/leg position. Feet can be close to or apart from each other.
E and T stand with backs to each other and lean into the back of the partner. Legs are shoulder-width apart. Bend the legs to parallel squat or deeper. Return to the starting position without pausing.	For this exercise E and T should be of approximately the same height and weight. E and T must bend the legs at the same time.	Different body/leg position. Feet can be close to each other or apart from each other. **PARTNER BALL SQUAT** Same exercise. Exercisers have big stability ball between their backs. Lean the back into the ball to keep it in place.
E and T standing side by side, both facing forward. Hand on the shoulder of the partner. Legs are shoulder-width apart. Bend the legs to parallel squat or deeper. Return to starting position without pausing. Both presses down with the arm to create resistance	For intermediate exercisers without knee problems. For this exercise E and T should be of approximately the same height and weight. E and T must bend the legs at the same time.	Different body/leg position. Feet can be close to each other or apart from each other.
E standing on one leg with the opposite leg lifted a little in front of the supporting leg. T stands by the side of E ready to support if necessary. E bends the leg as much as possible with the heel of the working leg on the floor. Return to the starting position without pausing.	For advanced exercisers without knee problems. Keep the foot on the floor to keep the knee stable.	Different arm/the body position. May be performed without a partner. Support on a wall bar. **STORK PRESS** Same exercise with the free leg lifted and held in horizontal throughout the exercise.

EXERCISE	TECHNIQUE

**SQUAT
STANDING WITH PARTNER
ON THE BACK**

Primary muscles:
Quadriceps,
gluteus maximus, hamstrings

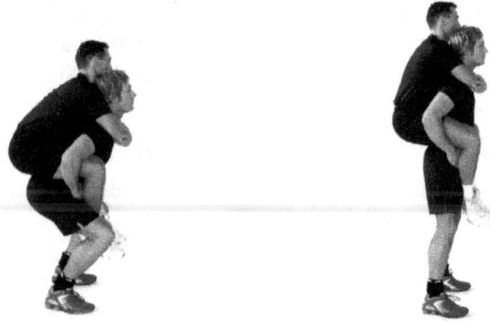

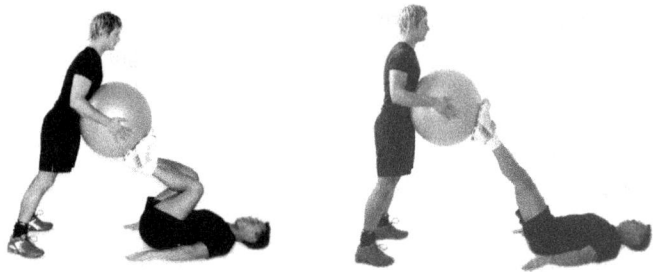

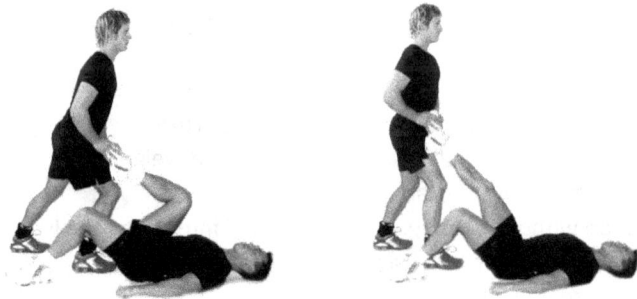

**LEG PRESS
SUPINE**

Primary muscles:
Quadriceps,
gluteus maximus, hamstrings

**SINGLE LEG PRESS
SUPINE**

Primary muscles:
Quadriceps,
gluteus maximus, hamstrings

**HAMSTRING CURL
PRONE**

Primary muscles:
Hamstrings

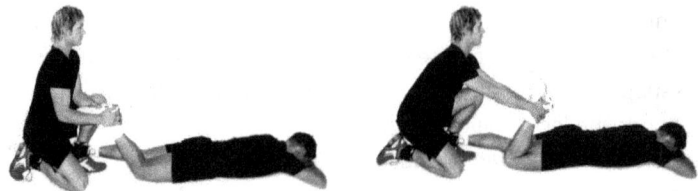

E standing. Feet shoulder-width apart. T sitting on the back of E with the legs around the waist of E. E bends the legs, squats down. Return to the starting position.	For advanced exercisers without back- or knee problems.	Different leg position.
E supine. Legs are bent and against the hips of T – or ball, as shown on the photo. E extends the legs and pushes T away. E bends the legs and lower T (and ball) with control.	The knees must bend without twisting; be careful that the bodyweight of T does not overload or twist the knees of E. The knees and feet should be aligned at all times.	Different leg angle. E's feet may rest on the hips of T or on a stability ball held by T.
E supine. One leg is bent or straight and on the floor. The other is flexed and on the hip of T. T stands with the feet staggered and leaning slightly on the leg of E. E extends the leg and pushes T away. E bends the leg and return with control.	The knee must bend without twisting; be careful that the bodyweight of T does not overload or twist the knee of E. The knee and foot should be aligned at all times.	Different leg angle.
E prone with one leg straight and relaxed. The other, working, leg is sligthly bent. T holds the hands on the heel or lower leg of E. E bends the leg as much as possible, while T resists. Resist the return movement.	The trainer or partner creates resistance, but must not push too hard. It may be necessary for partner to hold down thigh of the working leg.	On floor or bench. The thigh of the active leg may be on the floor or lifted a little into hip extension.

EXERCISE	TECHNIQUE

**NORDIC HAMSTRING CURL
KNEELING**

Primary muscles:
Hamstrings, gluteus maximus,
gastrocnemeus

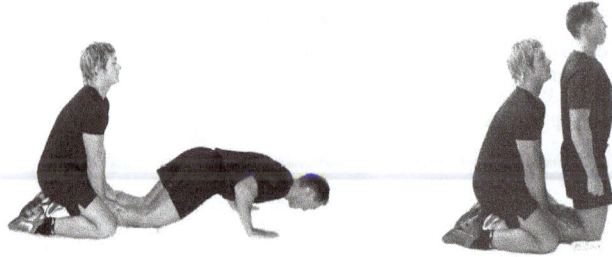

**LEG EXTENSION
PRONE**

Primary muscles:
Quadriceps

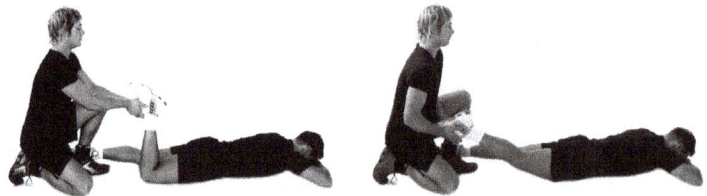

**HEEL RAISE
(DONKEY RAISE)
STANDING**

Primary muscles:
Gastrocnemeus, soleus

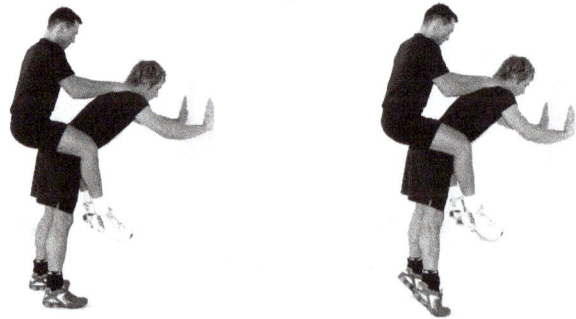

**TOE PULL
SITTING**

Primary muscles:
Tibialis anterior

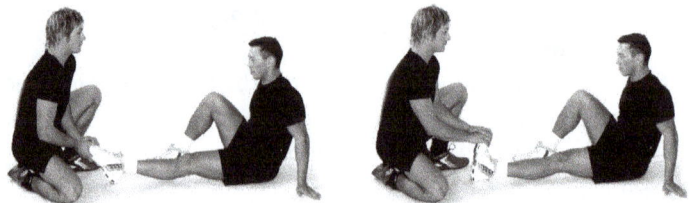

E kneeling. The torso erect. Arms relaxed. Feet anchored by T or a wall bar. E contracts the hamstrings and lowers the body, legs and torso, towards the floor. Stop before resting. E contracts the hamstrings and return the legs and torso close to vertical position.	For advanced exercisers. Excellent functional, but hard exercise. Put a mat under the lower legs, so the kneecaps are off the floor. This is more comfortable.	Different body/leg angle.
E prone with one leg straight. The other, working, leg is bent. T holds the hands on the shins of E. E extends knee, pushes lower leg down against resistance of T. Resist the return movement.	The trainer or partner creates resistance, but must not push too hard. It may be necessary for partner to hold down high of the working leg.	On floor or bench. Put a mat under the lower legs, so the kneecaps are off the floor. This is more comfortable.
E standing and leaning forward supporting hands on a wall or wall bar. T sits on the hips of E. E raises the heels and the body by contracting the calves. Lower with control.	Can be performed standing on a bench with the feet off the edge, but be careful not to go too low and overstretch the Achilles tendon.	With straight knees: Focus on gastrocnemeus With bent knees: Focus on soleus
E sitting with one leg bent and the other leg, the working leg, straight. T sits by the feet and holds the hands around the foot of E. E pulls the toes towards the shin, dorsiflexion, while T resists the movement. Resist the return movement.	The trainer or partner creates resistance, but must not push too hard.	Different body position – does not affect exercise.

EXERCISE	TECHNIQUE

**LEG ABDUCTION,
SIDELYING**

Primary muscles:
Gluteus medius and minimus

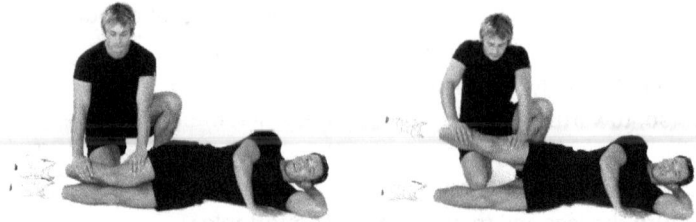

**LEG ADDUCTION,
SITTING**

Primary muscles:
Adductors

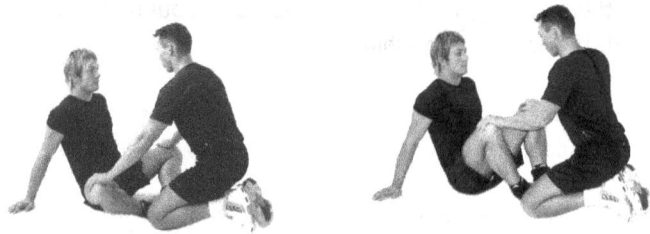

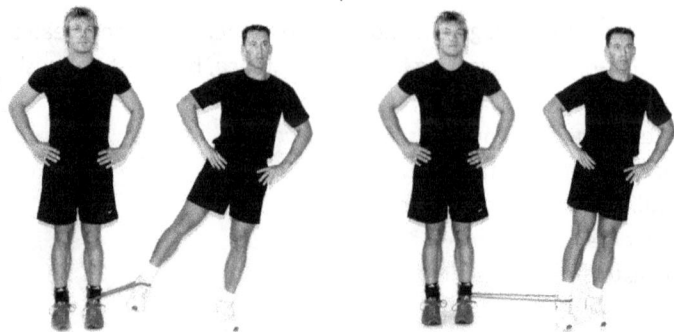

**ABDUCTION/ADDUCTION,
STANDING/SUPINE**

Primary muscles:
Gluteus medius and minimus,
adductors

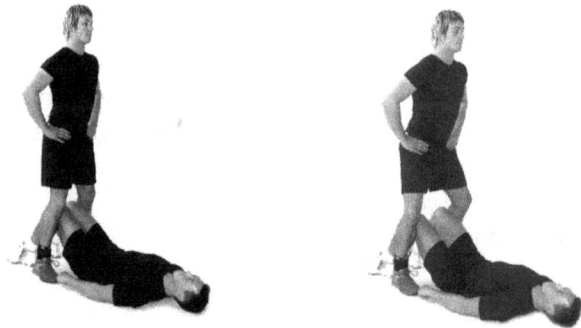

**LEG ADDUCTION, STANDING
WITH PARTNER
AND RUBBER BAND**

Primary muscles:
Adductors

E sidelying with body on a straight line. Top arm stabilizes the body. T kneels behind E and holdes the hands on the outer thigh and lower leg. E lifts, abducts, the top leg, while T resists the movement. T pushes the leg of E down, while E resists.	Contract the core muscles to stabilize the body to stabilize the body. T holds above and below the knee, not directly on the knee.	Hips flexed or straight. Knees bent or straight.
E sitting with feet together and bent legs with knees to the sides. T kneels by the feet and pushes the hands down on the inner thighs of E. E adducts the legs, while T resists the movement.	Be careful during this exercise. The exerciser must be ready and the trainer must not exert too much pressure to avoid straining adductor muscles.	Different leg position/angle.
E supine. Legs are bent, feet on the floor and together. T standing, legs slightly bent, feet on either side of the legs (outer thighs) of E. E abducts the legs, while T adducts. After a set change places, so T is supine and abducts and E is standing and adducts legs.	In this exercise both partners are active performing different exercises.	Different leg position. **AD/ABDUCTION SITTING** U and T sitting opposite each other. Legs straight or bent. E: Lower legs are on the out-side of the lower legs of T. E adducts, T abducts, resists. After a set change, so E abducts and T adducts.
E and T standing side by side. Both facing forward. E has a rubberband around the ankle anchored around the ankle of T. The working leg of E is to the side, abducted. T is a passive partner. E adducts the leg to the opposite leg. Resist the return movement. After a set change to the opposite leg.	Contract the core muscles to stabilize the body to stabilize Iron. Check the rubberband before starting.	Different angle – with internal or external rotation of the leg. From the front or the back (see Hip and Leg Exercises).

**AB CURL
WITH TUBE BACK TO BACK
SUPINE**

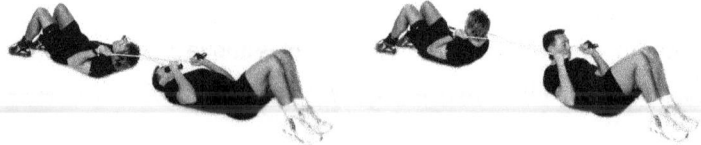

Primary muscles:
Rectus abdominis,
obliques externus and internus

**AB CURL
FEET AGAINST FEET
SUPINE**

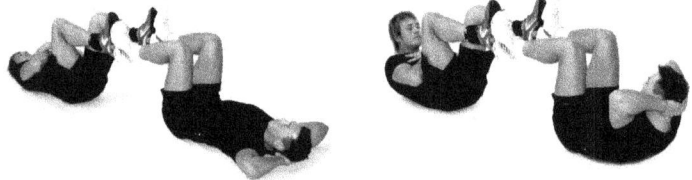

Primary muscles:
Rectus abdominis,
obliques externus and internus

**AB CURL
SUPINE WITH LEG SUPPORT**

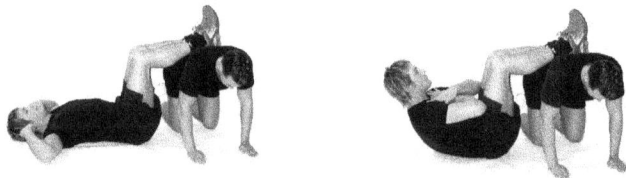

Primary muscles:
Rectus abdominis,
obliques externus and internus

**LEG CIRCLES
SITTING**

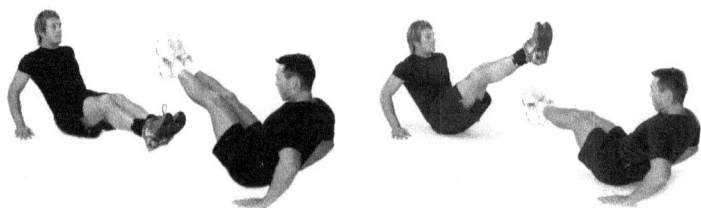

Primary muscles:
Rectus abdominis,
obliques externus and
internus, transversus
abdominis

E and T supine facing away from each other, approx. 7 ft, 2 m apart. The tubes are looped around each other and anchored by the hands by the shoulders. Both curl up the torso at the same time and speed. Lower with control.	Both curl up the torso at the same time. Check the tubing before starting.	**OBLIQUE CURL** **WITH RUBBERBAND** Same exercise with rotation left and right.
E and T supine. Legs bent 90 degrees in the hips and knees, tabletop position, with the feet against each other. Contract ab muscles to curl up the torso. Both curl up at the same time and speed. Lower with control.	Both exercisers are active in this exercise. The exercise can be performed without a partner with the feet up against a wall.	Different arm/leg position.
E supine with the legs across the back of T. Hands by the side of the head or at the chest. Contract ab muscles to curl up the torso. Lower with control.	One partner is passive. The exercise can be performed without a partner with the legs on a chair or bench.	Different arm position. Both partners can be active, if one performs a plank, while the partner performs ab curls.
E and T sitting opposite each other. Hands on the floor behind the body. Legs are straight and lifted. E and T circle legs around each others legs.	For advanced exercisers. Contract the core muscles to stabilize the body to protect the back. The exercise can be performed without a partner.	Different arm position. Different leg position.

**TORSO ROTATION
WITH TUBE OR BAND
STANDING**

Primary muscles:
Obliques externus and internus

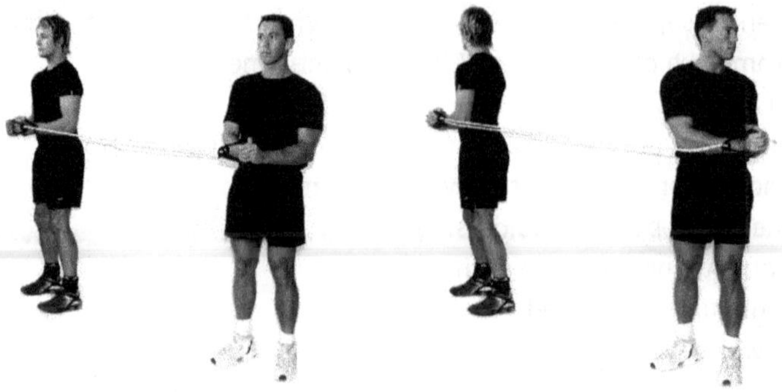

**REVERSE AB CURL
SUPINE**

Primary muscles:
Rectus abdominis,
obliques externus and internus

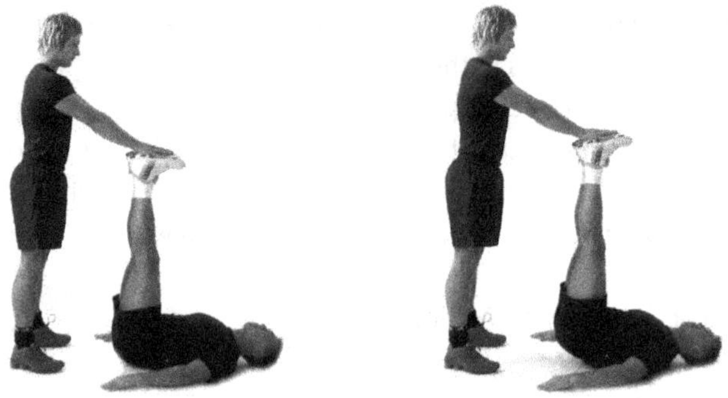

**LEGLIFT
SUPINE**

Primary muscles:
Rectus abdominis,
obliques externus and internus

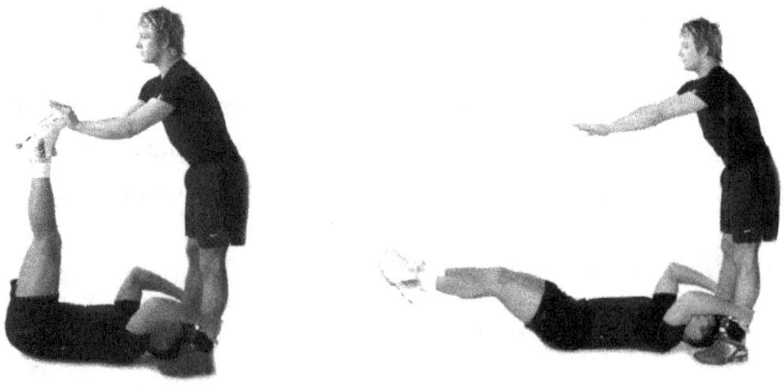

**AB CURL
HANGING FROM PARTNER**

Primary muscles:
Rectus abdominis, obliques
internus and externus,
transversus abdominis

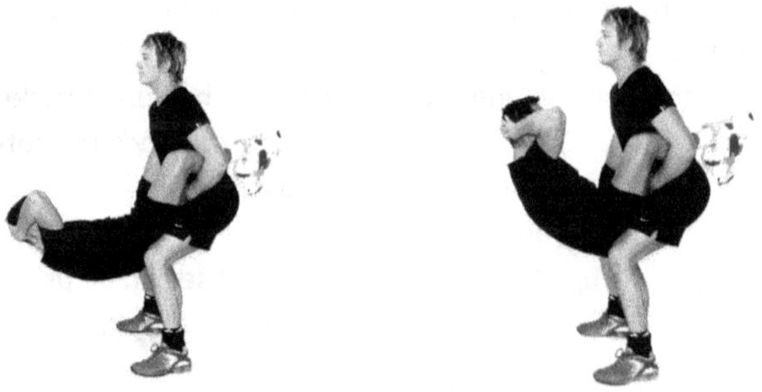

E and T standing side by side, both facing forward. Upper arms are close to the torso. Elbows bent, forearms in horizontal. Handles in hands. Tubes are looped around each other. Rotate torso out, away form the partner. After a set both face the other way. Repeat to the opposite side.	It is important that both exercisers pull at the same time. Feet, knees and hips must face the same way, forward. Rotation is from the navel and up. Avoid turning the hips. Check the tube before starting.	Different leg position.
E supine. Hips bent 90 degrees. Legs are straight and vertical. T stands and pushes down on the feet of E. E contracts the lower part of the abdominals to perform a pelvic tilt, to lift the legs up against the resistance. Lower with control.	Legs are straight or slightly bent, and vertical. The movement is in the lower part of the abdominals, not the hips.	Different leg position.
E supine. Hips bent 90 degrees. Legs are straight and vertical. T stands behind E. E holds on to lower legs of T to stabilize the body. E contracts the abdominals and lowers the legs to the floor and then lifts the legs up again. T pushes the legs back down, while E resists the movement.	For advanced exercisers. Contract the core muscles to stabilize the body to protect the lower back.	**DRAGON FLAGS** For very advanced exerciers: E lift the legs and the torso until only the upper back and shoulders are supporting. From this position lower torso and legs at the same time back to the starting position just above the floor.
E sitting/hanging with the legs around the waist of T. T stands with feet wide apart and torso erect and holds the legs of E. E contracts the abdominal muscles and curl up the torso. Lower with control.	For advanced exercisers. Important that T contracts the core muscles and keeps the torso as erect as possible.	Different arm position. **REVERSE AB CURL HANGING FROM PARTNER** One partner leans forward. The other supine on the back, holding the shoulders for support. Perform a reverse ab curl.

EXERCISE	TECHNIQUE

**WHEELBARROW
PLANK POSITION**

Primary muscles:
Rectus abdominis, obliques,
transversus abdominis, multifidii, shoulder- and
armmuscles

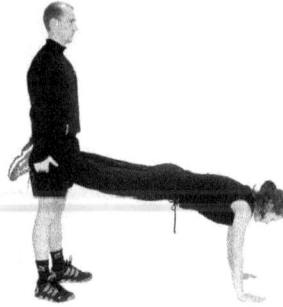

**REVERSE WHEELBARROW
BRIDGE POSITION**

Primary muscles:
Gluteus maximus, erector
spinae, the shoulder- and
arm muscles, transversus
abdominis, multifidii

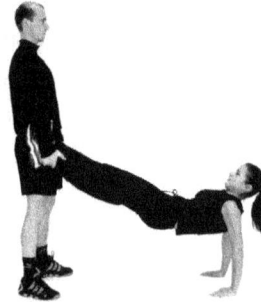

**SIDEPLANK
SUPPORTED BY PARTNER**

Primary muscles:
Quadratus lumborum,
transversus abdominis,
multifidii, obliques,
shoulder- and armmuscles

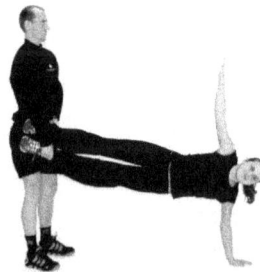

**BALANCE ON EXERCISE
BALL WITH
PARTNER PUSHING**

Primary muscles:
Transversus abdominis,
multifidii

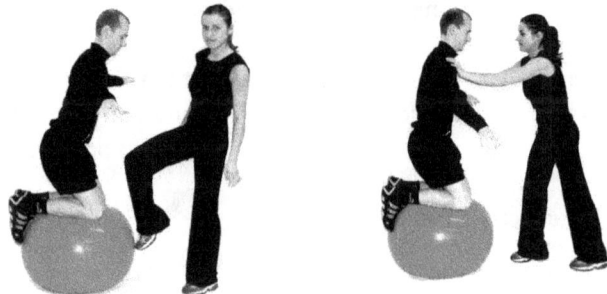

E in plank position, supporting on the hands. Body straight, neck in line with the spine. Core muscles contracted. T holds the lower legs of E. T walks around with E, like a 'wheelbarrow'. The body should not pike or sag.	Remember to keep breathing. Excellent core exercise with an element of play. Moderate tempo in order to protect the wrists.	You can walk forward, backward and to the side, so the exercise changes.
E in bridge position, supporting on the hands. Body as straight as possible. Buttocks are contracted to keep the bridge position. T holds the lower legs of E. T walks around with E, like a 'wheelbarrow' (reverse). The body should not sag.	Remember to keep breathing. Excellent core exercise with an element of play. Moderate tempo in order to protect the wrists.	You can walk forward, backward and to the side, so the exercise changes.
E in side plank position. Body is on a straight line with the core muscles contracted. Support on the bottom hand. T holds the lower legs of E. T carefully moves the legs forward, backwards, upwards and downwards.	The exercise can be performed without a partner with the feet anchored by a wall bar. Excellent core exercise with an element of play. Moderate tempo in order to protect the wrists and the shoulders.	Different arm position.
E is kneeling on a stability ball. T tries to make E loose the balance by kicking lightly to the ball or pushing the upper body of E. Various movements.	For balance, stability and coordination.	Different body/leg position. On top of the stability ball you can perform sports specific exercises, tennis serve, golf swing, handball throw, etc.

EXERCISE	TECHNIQUE

**AB CURL
WITH MEDICINE BALL AND HIP
ADDUCTION**

Primary muscles:
Rectus abdominis, obliques
externus and internus,
transversus abd., multifidii

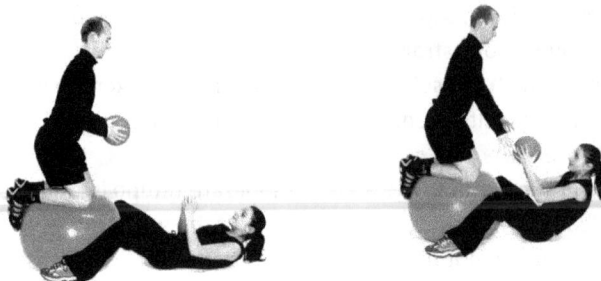

**SIDEBEND, LOWER BACK
SIDELYING
LEGS ANCHORED**

Primary muscles:
Quadratus lumborum

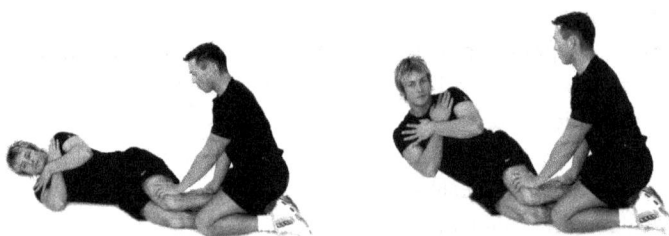

**EXTENSION AND FLEXION
WITH MEDICINE BALL
STANDING**

Primary muscles:
Erector spinae,
rectus abdominis

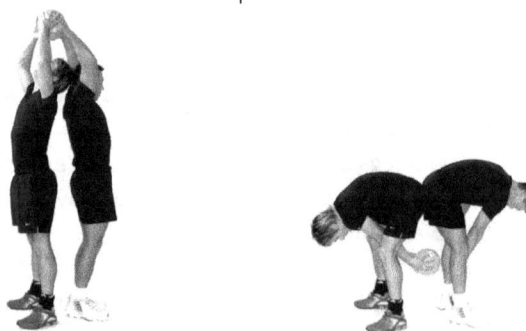

**TORSO ROTATION
STANDING
WITH MEDICINE BALL**

Primary muscles:
Obliques externus and
internus, rotators, multifidii

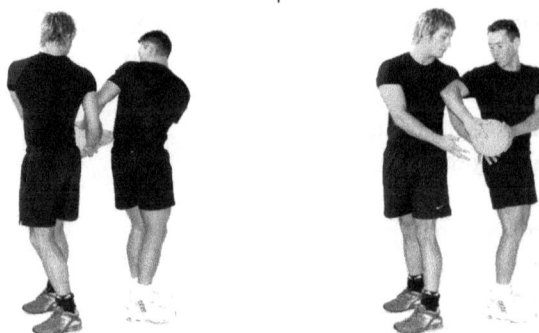

T is kneeling on a stability ball with a medicine ball in the hands. E supine with the legs apart and squeezing the ball, adduction. T leans forward with the ball. E curls up the torso and gets the ball in the top position. Lower. Curl up again and pass back ball to T. T extends the back. Repeat.	For coordination. Stability work for E. Strength training for the abdominal muscles and adductors for T.	Different leg position. A medicine ball is the preferred piece of equipment, but you may also use other balls.
E sidelying with legs slightly bent. The arms on the chest or behind the head. T sitting on the lower legs of E stabilizing the body. E sidebends and lifts the torso from the floor in the frontal plane. Lower with control. Do not pause. Repeat.	The exercise can be performed without a partner with the feet anchored by a wall bar.	Different arm position.
E and T stand back to back. E holds a medicine ball in the hands. E extends the arms overhead and passes the ball to T. T bends down and passes the ball to E between the legs. After one set, change direction and pass the ball the opposite way around.	Standing extension and flexion exercises are functional.	Different leg position. A medicine ball/ball is the preferred piece of equipment, but you may also use a dumbbell or kettlebell.
E and T stand back to back. E holds a medicine ball in the hands. E rotates the torso and passes the ball to T. T takes the ball and rotates to the other side to pass the ball back to E. After one set, change direction and pass the ball the opposite way around.	Standing rotation exercises are functional.	Different leg position. A medicine ball/ball is the preferred piece of equipment, but you may also use a dumbbell or kettlebell.

References

Aagaard, M (2006), *Aerobic – Functional Group Exercise*, Aagaard

Aagaard, M (2009), *Fitness og styrketræning*, Aagaard

Aagaard, M (2003), *Workout*, Aagaard

ACE (2000), *Group Fitness Instructor Manual*, ACE

ACE (2004), *Group Strength Training*, ACE

Baechle, TR, Earle, R (2000*), Essentials of Strength Training And Conditioning*, Human Kinetics

Baechle, TR, Groves, B R (1998), Weight *Training Steps to Success 2nd Ed.*, Human Kinetics

Bierring, F, Garby, L (1990), *Anatomi & Fysiologi*, Munksgaard

Boyle, M (2004), *Functional Conditioning for Sports*, Human Kinetics

Chek, PW (2000), *Chek Marks for Success,* CHEK Institute

Chek, PW (2002*), Chek Marks for Success II*, CHEK Institute

Chek, PW (2000), *Movement that matters*, CHEK Institute

Cibrario, M (1997*), Resistance exercises*, SPRI Products, Inc.

Delavier, F (2001, *Strength Training Anatomy*, Human Kinetics

DIF (2005*), Muskeltraening*, DIF

Gjerset et al. (2002*), Idraettens Traeningslaere, 2nd Ed.*, G.E.C. Gad

Gotved, H (1994*), Det er din krop*, Munksgaard

Gotved, H (1977), *Ha' det bedre. Kropserfaring*, P. Haase & Søns forlag

Kinakin, K (2006), *Optimal Muscle Training*, Human Kinetics

Mejdevi, M (1996*), En bog om grundtraening*, SISU Idrottsböcker

Peterson, L, Renström, P (1999), *Idraetsskader Idraetstraening,* Gyldendal

Schwarzenegger, A (1987), *Encyclopedia of Modern Bodybuilding*, Fireside

Simonsen, O, Larsen, A S, Kaalund, S (1995), *All-Round Fitness*, Centrum

Weismann, K (1995), *Muskeloversigt*, F.A.D.L.s Forlag

Wirhed, R (2006), *Anatomi & bevaegeseslaere i draet*, Duo

Zacho, M (2001), *Styrketraening*, DIF

Zatsiorsky, VM (1995), *Science and Practice of Strength Training*, Human Kinetics

Glossary

Ab curl	Flexion of the spine, exercise.
Abduction	Away from the midline of the body.
Adduction	Towards the midline of the body.
Agonist	The primary working muscle of the movement.
Antagonist	The muscle with the opposite function of the agonist.
Anterior	Nearer the front.
Barbell	Bar for weight plates.
Bent-over	Leaning forward, forward flexion (rows, etc.).
Bilateral	With both arms or legs.
Circumduktion	Circular movement.
Closed-chain	Training with distal segment anchored.
Concentric	Muscle contraction, the muscle shortens.
Contraction	Muscle work, the muscle shortens or lengthens.
Continuus	Action carries on without stopping or interruption.
Coordination	Neuro-muscular function.
Core training	Working the muscles between the pelvic floor and the diaphragm.
Curl	Bend, flex.
Crunch	Ab curl with pelvis and torso curling up at the same time.
Decline	Lying at an angle with the head downwards.
Dorsal	Towards the back of the body, foot or hand.
Dumbbell	A small bar with weight plates.
Eccentric	Muscle contraction, the muscle lengthens.
Elevation	Lifting.
Eversion	Outward rotation, the sole of the foot outwards.
Extension	Straightening.
Flex	Bend. Contract muscle.
Flexion	Bending.
Flys	The arms in horizontal plane making an embracing movement.
Frontal plane	Plane from shoulder to shoulder, lateral movements.
Functional training	Any training that has a function for sports or every day living.
Horizontal plane	Plane transversing the body, also transversal plane.
Hyperextension	Extending further than neutral, normal, position.

Glossary

Incline	Lying at an angle with the head upwards.
Inversion	Inward rotation, the sole of the foot turns in.
Isometric	Muscle contraction without joint movement.
Lateral	To the side, away from the midline of the body.
Ligament	Strong tissue connecting bone to bone.
Lumbar	Concerning the lower part of the back/spine.
Lunge	Stepping forward or out, exercise.
Medial	Towards the midline of the body.
Open-chain	Training with the distal segment moving freely (not anchored).
Overload	Increased load for continued progression.
Palmar	Towards the palm of the hand.
Partial	Smaller, limited range of motion.
Plantar	Towards the sole of the foot.
Plié	Squat with legs wide apart.
Prone	Lying face down.
Pronated	Hands or feet turned inwards/downwards.
Posterior	Placed behind or at the back.
Plyometrics	Explosive strength training, focus on the speed component.
Pronation	Hands of feet turned inward/downward.
Repetition	One complete move, concentric and eccentric phase
Rotation	Turning around an axis (left, right, medially, laterally).
Resistance band	Long flat piece of rubberband for resistance training.
Sagittal plane	From the back to the front, movement forward/backward.
Sit-up	Abdominal curl with hip flexion (the body comes up to the legs).
Spotter	A helper, who observes and assists during strength training.
Squat	Bending the legs, lowering the body. A classic functional exercise.
Supine	Lying face up.
Supination	Hands or feet turned outward/upward.
Synergist	Muscle working together with the agonist to perform the movement.
Set	A number of repetitions performed in sequence without a pause.
Tube	Long round (approx. 1,2 m) piece of rubbertube for resistance training.
Unilateral	With one arm or leg at a time.

About the Author

Marina Aagaard, *Master of Fitness and Exercise,* part-time associate professor at Aalborg University, Sports, and former head of the Fitness Department at the Coaching Academy of Denmark, 1995-2010, National Coach of Aerobic Gymnastics and consultant to the Danish Gymnastics Federation, 1995-2008.

Before that she served as a regional aerobics manager and health club manager for the Form and Figur health club chain. From 1991-1998 she co-owned and managed the family health club, BodyTeria, Aarhus, as well as working as a consultant and lecturer at her company aagaard.

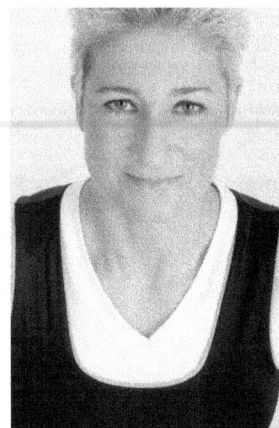

Marina is a certified Holistic Lifestyle Coach, CHEK Institute, and an American Council on Exercise certified group exercise instructor and personal trainer (gold).

For seven years she was head of the Danish Reebok Instructor Club and became a Step and Slide Reebok Master Trainer. Together with Gin Miller, the inventor of steptraining, she starred in the 1993-1994 Eurosport Step Reebok series.

At the same time Marina created and hosted her own morning aerobic TV-series as well as choreographing numerous aerobic and dance shows and performances for national television.

Her interest in elite training led to choreographing, coaching and judging at aerobics and fitness competions. Marina served as an Aerobic Gymnastics judge, Juge Breveté, for the FIG, the International Gymnastics Federation, and judged at every European and World Championship from 1995-2004.

For more than 25 years she has been involved in strength training and conditioning of recreational exercisers as well as world class athletes.

Marina has published numerous articles on fitness and is the author of a series of fitness books and more than 100 compendia on resistance training and group exercise.

Marina enjoys strength training, group exercise, running, skiing and skating as well as music, dance, art, cars and travelling. She and her husband, Henrik, reside in the bay area of Kalø Vig, Jutland, Denmark.

Fitness Books

Aerobic – Functional Group Exercise in Theory and Practice, 6th Ed.

344 pages

A bestselling book on all aspects of aerobics and group exercise in general.
Based on research and practical experience within all modalities of international group exercise, this text is a must for anyone working with group exercise. An indispensable manual on: Music, sound, choreography, teaching methods and organization.
Including a complete guide to aerobic and dance aerobic steps.

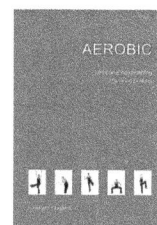

Step aerobics – four steps to optimal step training

264 pages, Danish

A popular textbook on everything you need to know about step training; the step, safety tips, correct stepping technique, various forms of step training. All about functional stepping – via intensity, impact and choreography.Including a comprehensive step guide, with more than 400 photos illustrating all basic steps and variations.

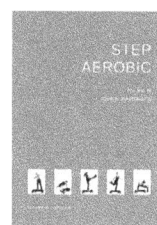

Workout – Group Resistance Training with Bodyweight or Equipment

235 pages, Danish

A popular textbook on resistance training, programmeming, exercises, sequencing and exercise technique. From isolation exercisesto complex, multi-exercises and functional training, for one-on-one and group resistance training, for beginning to advanced level. Designing workouts with bodyweight and equipment, including warm-up, balance work and core training. Including a comprehensive illustrated guide to exercises with bodyweight, barbells, dumbbells, tubes, bands, XerBars and UltraToners.

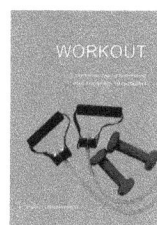

Spining, Biking & Cycling – Indoor Group Cycling in Theory and Practice

214 pages, Danish

An excellent handbook on one of the most popular forms of group exercise, group indoor cycling. For instructors and trainers. All about the indoor bike, setting up the bike, cycling equipment and riding technigue. Cardiovascular training and heart rate monitoring. In-depth descriptions of all parts of the group cycling class plus use of music and drills. Numerous ideas fordrills and teaching methods. Including 20 complete programmes.

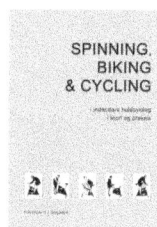

Resistance Training Exercises – Fitness and performance exercises

337 pages

The number one resource for resistance training exercises. It is all about exercises and variations. From simple isolations to advanced multi-exercisesfor one-on-one or group resistance training, for recreational or Olympic athletes.
With bodyweight, dumbbells, barbells, rubberbands,, tubes and bands. Also a great section on partner exercises. Comprehensive tables of more than 400 exercises, illustrated with over 800 photos plus descriptions and notes.

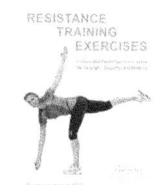

Stability Ball Exercises – Fitness and performance exercisess

358 pages

The number one resource for stability ball exercises for everyone using the stability ball; coaches, trainers, instructors, physiotherapists, chiropractors and PE teachers.
For one-on-one fitness, group exercise and sports and physical exercise, for recreational exercisers to Olympic class athletes. The book contains comprehensive tables of more than 450 exercises, illustrated with more than 900 photos plus descriptions and notes.

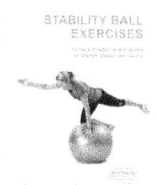

www.ingramcontent.com/pod-product-compliance
Lightning Source LLC
Chambersburg PA
CBHW081621280326
41928CB00055B/2878